the **facts**
Sexually
transmitted
infections

the **facts**

Sexually
transmitted
infections

THIRD EDITION

DR DAVID BARLOW MA, BM BCh, FRCP, FRCP (EDIN)

Consultant Physician, Department of Genitourinary
Medicine, Guy's and St Thomas' Foundation Trust
Honorary Fellow Sri Lanka College of Venereologists
Honorary Senior Lecturer London University

'HIV and AIDS – the clinical picture' with
DR JULIE FOX BSc, MB ChB, MRCP, MD
Consultant Physician, Department of Genitourinary
Medicine, Guy's and St Thomas' Foundation Trust

© Cartoons, Geoffrey Dickinson 1979

OXFORD
UNIVERSITY PRESS

OXFORD
UNIVERSITY PRESS

Great Clarendon Street, Oxford OX2 6DP

Oxford University Press is a department of the University of Oxford.
It furthers the University's objective of excellence in research, scholarship,
and education by publishing worldwide in

Oxford New York

Auckland Cape Town Dar es Salaam Hong Kong Karachi
Kuala Lumpur Madrid Melbourne Mexico City Nairobi
New Delhi Shanghai Taipei Toronto

With offices in

Argentina Austria Brazil Chile Czech Republic France Greece
Guatemala Hungary Italy Japan Poland Portugal Singapore
South Korea Switzerland Thailand Turkey Ukraine Vietnam

Oxford is a registered trade mark of Oxford University Press
in the UK and in certain other countries

Published in the United States
by Oxford University Press Inc., New York

© Oxford University Press 2011

The moral rights of the authors have been asserted
Database right Oxford University Press (maker)

First edition published 1979

Second edition published 2006

British Library Cataloguing in Publication Data

Data available

Library of Congress Cataloging in Publication Data

Typeset in Plantin
by Glyph International, Bangalore, India

Printed in Great Britain on acid-free paper by
Ashford Colour Press Ltd., Gosport, Hampshire

ISBN 978-0-19-959565-5

10 9 8 7 6 5 4 3 2 1

Reviews of earlier editions

This book is written in an approachable manner and makes enjoyable reading, getting across difficult concepts such as false-positives and false-negatives. Overall this book is a delight to read, offering patients a refreshingly balanced outlook on the diagnosis and management of infections. *International Journal of STD & AIDS*

Dr Barlow has written an excellent book, factual, short, and witty. The book is aimed at a wide audience and is desirable reading for all well-educated doctors. It is an important addition to the range of books available on the subject and contains a description of all the important issues in modern genitourinary medicine. *The Lancet*

This ought to be in every school and public library. Barlow has a great deal to teach all doctors. The author pays us the complement of writing in plain English: buy, borrow or steal it, you won't find my copy on the second-hand market. David Cargill, *World Medicine*

This book on sexually transmitted diseases will be of interest to a wide range of readers, including health educators and those in other health professions. Chapters on each of the infections contain a wealth of information. This book will be a welcome addition to libraries in schools, colleges for further education, teaching hospitals and medical group practices. *British Journal of Venereal Diseases*

Preface

Five years ago I sent off the final proofs of the second edition of this book. Since then there have been significant changes. *Mycoplasma genitalium* is established as a major cause of urethritis in men and equivalent infections in women.

We have seen the evolution of an extraordinary strain of *Chlamydia trachomatis* in Sweden, with its *invisibility cloak* enabling it to bypass our diagnostic tests and disappear from view.

Vaccination against HPV is now an established weapon against genital warts and cancer, and new management of HIV infection has reduced problems associated with treatment just as it has increased high-quality lifespan.

There is much that is new.

Readers may find that my advice or interpretation in certain areas differs from the standard. If in doubt, it is best to consult your local GUM clinic.

David Barlow
August 2010

Preface to 2ⁿᵈ Edition

The first edition of this volume was published 27 years ago and a multitude of changes has occurred since then. In 1979, while headlines talked of the 'love virus', as herpes was labelled, no one was aware that another more deadly virus was spreading rapidly and inexorably from central Africa via Haiti to the East and then West coasts of North America. Although infection with the human immunodeficiency virus (HIV) was not to be recognized for another two years (and not named as such for a further four), this 'silent' period, akin to the latent period of the virus itself, allowed an insidious, lethal infection to infiltrate and establish itself in its first Western target group, gay men.

Aside from HIV infection, incidence of the other sexually transmitted diseases has changed (invariably upward) and the emphasis has shifted from bacterial infections to viral ones, warranting separate chapters for genital herpes and genital warts in this new edition. We should wonder at the new drugs that have become available, easier to take, more effective and often with fewer side-effects. There are new antivirals, new antifungals and new antibacterial preparations, many, however, remaining beyond the budget of developing economies. We should also wonder at the new diagnostic tools that are used—a quick 'pee-and-go' urine test replacing the infamous 'bottle-brush' for chlamydial and gonococcal infections in men. However convenience may come at the price of false positives and negatives. A short chapter takes you through the pitfalls of interpreting these and other results.

Vaginal discharge, such a common symptom and still so often a source of misery, has yielded up some important secrets. In 1979, I wrote of 'non-specific vaginitis' caused by *Haemophilus vaginalis*. A year later this bacterium was renamed *Gardnerella vaginalis* while the condition briefly became 'anaerobic vaginosis' and then 'bacterial vaginosis' (BV) in the early 1980s. That decade witnessed the identification of the multitude of other bacteria responsible for the symptoms of BV and a better understanding of the factors that make this most common of conditions likely to occur and recur.

Our knowledge of Human Papilloma Virus infection (HPV), responsible for warts both plain and genital, has expanded along with the introduction of topical treatments that promise to lighten the clinical and personal load of managing this common infection. How common? New diagnostic tools, using techniques of molecular biology, demonstrate that a majority of sexually active

25-year-old women are already infected with HPV. Thankfully, most of them do not go on to develop clinical warts.

Human immunodeficiency virus is included because it is primarily a sexually transmitted condition but this book cannot provide a comprehensive review of HIV infection and AIDS; for that there are other reference sources. We can all learn from an understanding of how and why the disease spread in the way it did, and from the (slow) development of tolerance for those particularly affected. I am grateful to have had the assistance of Dr Ali Mears in writing the section on the medical aspects of HIV infection; she is an able and knowledgeable clinician.

In 1979, my clinic at St Thomas' Hospital coped with 12,000 attendances. In 2005, some 45,000 pairs of feet will cross our threshold but will endure waiting times as unacceptable today as they would have been unthinkable 26 years ago. Annual attendance at GUM clinics in the UK has trebled and we are currently witnessing a resurgence of the 'classical' venereal diseases, gonorrhoea and syphilis, as well as record new cases of chlamydial infection. In spite of which gloom, there is still available in Great Britain the best service for the diagnosis and treatment of sexually transmitted diseases to be found anywhere in the world.

I hope this new edition will put the disease prevalence in perspective and help those who have, or think they have, or want to know how to avoid, or even just wish to know more about, sexually transmitted diseases, to adopt a calm approach to what is, these days, an eminently manageable group of conditions.

David Barlow London 2005

Contents

Abbreviations

AIDS	acquired immunodeficiency syndrome
BV	bacterial vaginosis
CDC	Centers for Disease Control
CIN	cervical intraepithelial neoplasia
GP	general practitioner
GPI	general paralysis of the insane
GU	genitourinary
GUM	genitourinary medicine
HAART	highly active antiretroviral therapy
HIV	human immunodeficiency virus
HPA	Health Protection Agency
HPV	human papilloma virus
HSV	herpes simplex virus
HVS	high vaginal swab
IDU	injecting drug users
IMB	intermenstrual bleeding
IUCD	intrauterine contraceptive device
LAP	lower abdominal pain
LGV	lymphogranuloma venereum
MC	*Molluscum contagiosum*
MG	*Mycoplasma genitalium*
MSM	men who have sex with men
MSU	mid-stream urine
NAAT	nucleic acid amplification tests
NGU	non-gonococcal urethritis
NNRTI	non-nucleoside reverse transcriptase inhibitor
NRTI	nucleoside reverse transcriptase inhibitor
NSGI	non-specific genital infection
NSU	non-specific urethritis
nvCT	new variant *Chlamydia trachomatis*
OI	opportunistic infection

PCP	*Pneumocystis carinii* pneumonia
PEP	post-exposure prophylaxis
PI	protease inhibitor
PID	pelvic inflammatory disease
SARA	sexually acquired reactive arthritis
STD	sexually transmitted disease
STI	sexually transmitted infection
TV	*Trichomonas vaginalis*
UTI	urinary tract infection
VD	venereal disease
VIN	vulval intraepithelial neoplasia
VVS	vulval vestibulitis syndrome

Acknowledgements

I am indebted to past and present colleagues at St Thomas' Hospital. I single out the late Dr Nicol Thin, eminent venereologist, critic, and good friend, and Dr James Bingham, long-standing friend and colleague.

Dr Ali Mears collaborated on the 'clinical aspects of HIV' chapter in the second edition, which has provided the template for this chapter. Ali has moved to a Consultant post elsewhere in London and I am pleased that Dr Julie Fox, a new Consultant colleague in our Trust, has agreed to contribute her considerable expertise as clinician and researcher in the field of HIV/AIDS.

My most important support comes from my wife Angela. Max and Sophie have joined Helena, Ella, and Francesca in the increasing list of grandchildren short-changed by my huddle over the keyboard.

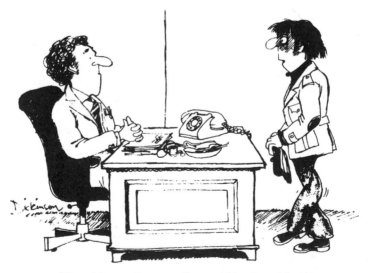

'It's not for me Doctor— I'm enquiring for a friend.'

1

Sexually transmitted infections—what to do

> ## Key points
>
> - Specialist sexual health clinics are found throughout the UK
> - Nearly every disease can be cured and *all* can be managed
> - Consultation and treatment are free and there is no need for a referral from a general practitioner (GP) or other doctor.

Where do I go?

The UK is one of three countries, with Ireland and Malta, which recognize management of sexually transmitted infections (STIs) as a separate medical specialty.

There is a network of over 250 genitourinary medicine (GUM) clinics in the UK, staffed by health professionals, including doctors, nurses, and health advisers. In other parts of the world, STIs are managed by different specialists—dermatovenereologists are the predominant providers of service in Europe, having expertise in skin conditions as well as STIs. One of the GUM clinics' more important roles is to *exclude* STIs, reassuring people that they are not infected. For example, the majority of human immunodeficiency virus (HIV) tests and results (most of which are negative) are given in GUM clinics.

What might I have caught?

'Germs' come in different sizes:

- A **virus** is so small that it can only survive and reproduce inside a living cell. Herpes simplex and the germs causing warts are viruses
- **Bacteria** are larger than viruses and most can survive away from their host and even multiply. *Treponema pallidum* and *Neisseria gonorrhoeae* are bacteria
- Next up in size come the **protozoa**, single-celled organisms like *Trichomonas vaginalis* (Chapter 3) or *Entamoeba histolytica* (Chapter 10)

◆ Larger still are the **parasites**, including *Phthirus pubis*, the crab louse, and *Sarcoptes scabiei*, which causes scabies.

Where to go for help?

The GP is ideally placed to advise those worried about the possibility of an STI. Most family practices will have a nurse with special training in sexual health who can help with questions of family planning, cervical smear tests, and STIs.

The *upside* of the GP consultation is that you are dealing with a familiar face who knows your health background, in familiar surroundings, conveniently situated. The *downside* is that you are dealing with a familiar face who probably knows the rest of your family and may even be a family friend. You may not wish to share your problem under these circumstances.

What about a GUM clinic?

The emphasis in a genitourinary (GU) clinic is on discretion. In the bad old days, the 'special' clinic was hidden, often in a basement, and decidedly away from the main, 'nice' parts of the hospital. Nowadays, the GUM clinic is designed and run to respect and maintain confidentiality, and most are found within the main body of the hospital.

All doctors are bound by a duty of confidentiality but this has extra force in GUM clinics, enshrined by an Act of Parliament incorporating the 'NHS Trusts and Primary Care Trusts (Sexually transmitted Diseases) Directions 2000'. Phew! I quote:

> Every…Trust shall take all necessary steps to secure that any information capable of identifying an individual obtained by any of their members or employees with respect to persons examined or treated for any sexually transmitted disease shall not be disclosed except [and I paraphrase] to another health care professional also involved in their care or to prevent spread.

The key word in clinics is CONFIDENTIALITY!

So, your details and the details of any infections are safeguarded by law. Even attendance at a clinic is kept secret, so the innocent telephone call, 'Can I have a word with my wife, Mrs Smith—I know she's there?', will be answered with a negative that neither acknowledges Mrs Smith's presence nor whether she is a patient at the clinic; patient records are even kept separately from the ordinary hospital notes.

This is one of the reasons that people with HIV infection in the UK have preferred to be looked after by GU physicians, for both outpatient and inpatient care.

You will be asked for personal details, including name, date of birth, and address. It is quite acceptable to insist on no contact at home and some attenders simply fail to give any address and give a false name. That is fine as long as the patient remembers what name they have given. In our department we have over 300 'John Smiths', some of them no doubt genuine, 15 'Mickey Mouses', and a round dozen 'Donald Ducks'.

The other advantages of attending a clinic are:

- Personnel—even in the smallest clinic there will be a specialist nurse and health adviser as well as the doctor, and there is usually a larger team whose combined expertise cannot be achieved in other settings
- Investigations—there will be a larger range of tests than is feasible at a GP's surgery
- Diagnostic facilities—because some samples can be examined on site, the correct diagnosis and treatment may be available at the time of first attendance.

Gonorrhoea, syphilis, non-specific urethritis (NSU), thrush, bacterial vaginosis, and *Trichomonas vaginalis* are all diagnosable on the spot, although the success rate of instant diagnosis does vary.

Finding other people who may also be infected (contact tracing) is a crucial part of the work of a GUM clinic, and 'partner notification' is handled sensitively as a cooperation between patients and clinic staff.

What investigations will I have?

There is a list of standard tests that are done for those who attend 'just for a check-up', including blood for syphilis and HIV (one sample does for both tests). All comers are tested for chlamydial infection and gonorrhoea, and women will usually have samples looked at for three vaginal conditions: thrush, bacterial vaginosis, and *Trichomonas vaginalis*.

Someone might take the above set of tests before embarking on a new sexual relationship. Other tests, including more specialized ones for syphilis or herpes, are not routine but will be done if indicated by clinical findings or a patient's story. Usually a woman's urine will be tested and a mid-stream urine sample (MSU) sent off if a urinary tract infection (UTI) is suspected.

In larger GUM departments there will be clinics for:

- Smear tests (cervical cytology) and colposcopy (Chapter 8)
- Psychosexual problems
- Contraception
- Genital skin conditions
- Other specialist problems.

Gay men attending a clinic have their own sets of tests because some infections are found more often than in straight people. For instance, tests for hepatitis A and B (Chapter 11) will be routine unless there is a good history of vaccination.

What if I am too young?

There are no restrictions on age, at either end of the scale, although the *very* young will, for obvious reasons, be accompanied by a parent or guardian. Those under the age of consent, 16 in the UK, do not need to have an older relative present and their confidentiality will be respected just like anyone else who attends.

What happens when I attend a GUM clinic?

Some clinics maintain an open-access, no-appointment system, which can mean longer waiting times but does guarantee same-day consultation once (and if) registration has taken place. Clinics with appointment systems will still see people whose problem is an emergency ('my (*now ex-*) partner says he has given me gonorrhoea') on the same day.

UK clinics are pledged to see new patients within 48 hours

In some clinics there are different locations or times for the different sexes, while in others there is a common waiting area. After registering, there may be 'triage' in which the special needs of each patient are assessed and they are then channelled towards, say, a quick screening service or a slower medical assessment.

Who do I talk to?

The medical history is usually taken by a doctor or, increasingly these days, a nurse practitioner or nurse consultant. Whichever it is, you must understand that they have 'heard it all before'. For many people this will be the first time they have talked seriously about sex with anyone. Shame, embarrassment, anger, and guilt, all may influence a patient's attitude to the consultation. Try to remember that when you are asked a particularly personal question it is not idle curiosity that prompts the question.

What happens to a woman in a GUM clinic?

Once the history has been taken, including menstrual and obstetric history, you will be offered an examination. This starts with a look at the vulva and pubic region and usually includes passing a speculum into the vagina. The prospect of this examination seems to fill many women with terror but, if done gently and slowly, there is no need for discomfort or pain; it does help if the woman is relaxed.

The Cusco's speculum is the most commonly used instrument. It has two, unfortunately named, 'blades' hinged at one end and is oval or vulva-shaped at the other. It is common practice to turn the speculum through 90° once inserted, before opening the two halves. The entrance to the vagina is designed to receive a cylindrical object, the penis, and it has always surprised me that this uncomfortable twisting movement remains standard practice.

Cusco designed his speculum to be used with the handles between the buttocks, which is more comfortable than with the handle by the clitoris. The thoughtful operator will make sure that the wider, outside, end of the speculum is warm, as well as the blades. Disposable plastic speculums do not need warming.

Where do they take samples from?

Samples are taken with a cotton-tipped swab from the vagina and the cervix, and are then examined using the microscope or sent off to the laboratory for culture or other forms of identification. 'Taking a sample' sounds as if it might be painful or uncomfortable. It isn't. Try rubbing a cotton bud gently across the back of your hand and that will reproduce exactly the pressure and feeling. Increasingly, women are encouraged to take their own samples.

If gonorrhoea is being excluded, samples will need to be taken from the urethra and rectum in women. Rectal-positive cases do not necessarily result from rectal intercourse (although they might), as gonorrhoea can find its way into the back passage as a result of general moistness of the area and gravity. Neither urethral nor rectal samples are painful, but are described as 'feeling a bit strange'.

What is a bimanual examination?

After the speculum examination, a bimanual examination may follow. This is particularly important if there is a story of pain in the pelvic area, lower abdomen, or deep pain during intercourse. In a bimanual examination, one or two fingers of one hand are inserted into the vagina while the other, usually left, hand feels the lower abdomen (hence *bimanual*, two hands). In this way, the doctor can look for evidence of pelvic inflammatory disease, fibroids, or see whether the uterus is enlarged if pregnancy is suspected.

The patient waits while the various samples are microscopically examined. Vaginal discharge, itching, or smell are most easily diagnosed on the spot. Gonorrhoea, if present, is found in less than half of cases (the others being diagnosed after culture in the laboratory).

If the tests are negative at the time of the initial examination, it is a good idea to ask the doctor whether there is likely to be any infection or what has caused your symptoms. The important thing to remember is that a definite diagnosis cannot be made until the laboratory investigations have been completed and the fact that nothing has been found *at the time* of the first visit does not mean that there is no infection.

What happens to a man in a GUM clinic?

A man's progression through the clinic differs only in detail from that of the woman. Like a woman, a man will be asked about his recent sexual encounters and whether a condom was used. Questions regarding a partner's origin might appear intrusive, but such information can be vital when deciding on treatment. Gonorrhoea from the Philippines is less easy to manage than gonorrhoea from Philadelphia.

After the history, the doctor will want to examine the penis and, if relevant, the anus, for sores, spots, swellings, or evidence of discharge. The foreskin will be pulled back in the uncircumcised man to look for signs on the glans or the inside of the foreskin for warts. The scrotum will be examined: testes, epididymis, and cords, often the only time a man has this sort of examination. Ideally a man should examine his testicles regularly for unusual lumps, just as a woman should her breasts.

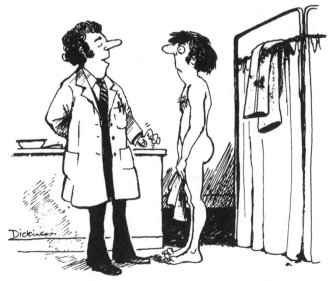

'I'm afraid I've got some bad news for your friend'.

Tests for chlamydia and gonorrhoea can be performed these days simply on a sample of urine. Such screening tests are fine because they are sensitive and will usually pick up infection if it is there. There may be problems with false positives (Chapter 2) and they do not pick up non-chlamydial urethritis, NSU, a common diagnosis made in men attending the GUM clinic. To diagnose NSU and gonorrhoea on the spot, a urethral sample needs to be taken.

Why am I asked not to urinate before attending?

The urethra is a rich source of diagnostic material and, since urinating tends to wash out the urethra, it helps if the patient has held his urine for at least 3 hours.

A thin plastic loop is gently inserted 2 cm into the urethra and any discharge examined with the microscope. Part of the discharge is sent to the laboratory. If rectal intercourse has taken place, samples will also be taken from the rectum for microscopy and culture.

> In general, men are more likely than women to leave the clinic with a diagnosis at the end of their first visit

If syphilis is suspected, a special microscopic examination is performed on fluid from a sore or rash.

What if I have HIV infection?

The majority of people who come to the clinic do not have HIV infection, so nearly all the HIV tests performed are negative. In the UK (Chapter 12), those most at risk of HIV infection are gay men and heterosexual men or women from sub-Saharan Africa. HIV-positive injecting drug users (IDUs) are rare these days. At the time of writing (mid-2010), there is not a significant amount of transmission of HIV occurring in this country between heterosexuals.

Whatever your sexual orientation, geographical origin, or colour, there is one certainty in the UK: *it is better to test for HIV than not to test.* Chapter 13 goes into the reasons but, in essence, today's management is so much better than previously that HIV infection can be controlled in virtually all cases– **but only once the diagnosis has been made.**

All GUM clinics have facilities for HIV testing and experienced staff to explain all the processes. The message is simple: if in doubt, test! Increasingly, a 'point-of-care' HIV test is available with a provisional result the same day.

How can I use this book to find out if I have an infection?

The quick answer is to follow my advice and pop down to your local clinic and clear the matter up, once and for all. But, in real life, you want an answer now, so the following might point you towards a likely, or at least possible, diagnosis without having to leave your armchair.

The list of infections passed on by or during sexual activity seems to grow year by year. While it is true that an even larger number of diseases can be passed on by close proximity with an infected person—for instance, the common cold or tuberculosis—no one would claim these as predominantly sexually transmitted. However, common sense (and medical experience) suggests that if, having had sex with someone with a cold, you start to sneeze and sniffle, it is more likely to be a cold than chlamydia.

As you read this book, you will find out how different infections vary in their ability to cause symptoms and how, in many people, there may be no symptoms at all. In general, women come off worse than men in this respect, more often showing no signs or symptoms of their disease. None the less, there are some symptoms that do give clues to their cause.

Women's symptoms

Itching and vaginal discharge are both dealt with in Chapter 3 (page 23), with candida being the most common cause. Itching around the vulva is also sometimes seen in genital herpes (Chapter 7, page 65) and genital warts (Chapter 8, page 72).

Vaginal odour is dealt with in Chapter 3. A bad smell is usually caused by bacterial vaginosis (page 25), less commonly *Trichomonas vaginalis* (page 28), and, rarely, a retained tampon (page 29).

Dysuria (stinging or burning when passing urine) in women is often caused by a urinary tract infection (UTI—see end of chapter), but is very occasionally seen with chlamydial infection (Chapter 5, page 49) or gonorrhoea (Chapter 4, page 39). If the pain comes when urine passes over sore patches outside on the vulva, an 'external' dysuria, then thrush or, rarely, herpes may be the cause, in which case there may be difficulty, as well as pain, in passing urine. UTIs may provoke frequency of urination, noticeable particularly at night.

Unusual vaginal bleeding will more often be caused by a gynaecological or oral contraceptive-related problem. It is occasionally seen in chlamydial cervicitis (Chapter 5, page 50).

Lower abdominal pain (LAP) can be associated with chlamydial (Chapter 6, page 54) or gonococcal (Chapter 4, page 40) infection and chronic pain can be associated with adhesions (Chapter 6, page 55). There are many other causes, from endometriosis to food poisoning and cystitis to fibroids, and, rarely, ectopic pregnancy, none of them STIs.

Pain having sex broadly divides into two sorts.

- *'Deep' dyspareunia* results from the erect penis pushing against sensitive, tender, possibly infected, contents in the pelvis. As with LAP (see above), deep pain on intercourse may be due to gonorrhoea or chlamydia and the other causes of LAP

- *'Superficial' dyspareunia* describes pain on the vulva or at the entrance to the vagina and can be seen with thrush or *Trichomonas vaginalis* or herpes. Poor lubrication may lead to tightness and discomfort (Chapter 3, page 24).

Lumps or bumps on the genitalia—there is a list of the half dozen or so most common lumps and bumps in the section on warts (Chapter 8, page 74).

Ulcers on the genitalia may be caused by trauma, thrush or herpes, and (uncommonly in the UK or USA) the tropical diseases described in Chapter 10.

Men's symptoms

Lumps and bumps are, as in women, dealt with in the chapter on warts (Chapter 8, page 74).

Dysuria describes any discomfort when passing water, and was classically a symptom of gonorrhoea (Chapter 4, page 38) and NSU (Chapter 5, page 49). It is sometimes found with herpes, *Trichomonas vaginalis*, and thrush (Chapter 3, page 24), and rarely with a UTI.

Urethral discharge is found with gonorrhoea (Chapter 4, page 38) and chlamydia, mycoplasma genitalium, and NSU (Chapter 5, page 47), and, rarely, with a foreign body (Chapter 5, page 48). Like dysuria, it is sometimes found with herpes (Chapter 7), *Trichomonas vaginalis*, and thrush (Chapter 5, page 47).

Ulcers on the genitalia may be caused by trauma, thrush, particularly on the foreskin in uncircumcised men (Chapter 5, page 47) or herpes (Chapter 7, page 64) and, uncommonly in the UK or USA, the tropical diseases described in Chapter 10.

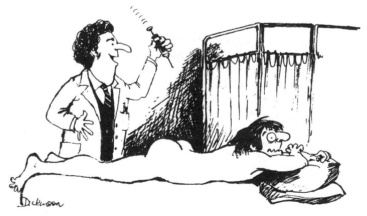

'This is going to hurt you more than your friend!'

Redness and/or itching of the glans penis are classical symptoms of thrush (Chapter 5, page 47), although small flat warts (Chapter 8, page 73) can give a similar appearance. Some skin conditions also give these symptoms.

Perianal itching in both sexes is usually caused by candidal infection (Chapter 3, page 24), although rectal gonorrhoea, when there may also be some discharge, can cause it (Chapter 4, page 39). Threadworms (Chapter 10, page 91) are another cause.

This is not an exhaustive list of possible symptoms and I have purposely not listed any that might be found with HIV infection or acquired immunodeficiency syndrome (AIDS). This is because they are often non-specific, such as headache or cough, and will virtually always be caused by something other than acquired immunodeficiency.

Urinary tract infections

I deal with these in this chapter because some of the symptoms of UTIs are shared with STIs, rather than because cystitis is sexually transmitted, which it isn't. However, symptoms similar to UTI may be brought on by intercourse, in what used (inaccurately) to be called 'honeymoon' cystitis. When this occurs there is no bacterial infection and the symptoms of dysuria and frequency are brought on because of poor vulval and vaginal lubrication. Better lubrication and peeing after sex cope with most cases.

Women are more prone to UTIs than men because of the closeness of the urethral opening, just above the vagina, to the anus, and the responsible bacteria are often the same as are found in the intestine. The classical symptoms are *dysuria* and *frequency*, particularly at night. There may be blood in the urine, *haematuria*, and *urgency*, a feeling of needing to go *now*.

Recurrent urine infections are not uncommon and are best sorted out by the GP, who can send urine samples (the MSU) to the laboratory to identify the bacteria and which antibiotics to use. Many people are unwilling to take antibiotics but, with UTIs, particularly if they keep recurring, failure to eradicate the germs may lead to spread into the kidneys with serious consequences.

Drinking plenty of fluids has always been a good suggestion. Cranberry juice is believed by many to ease the symptoms of cystitis but avoid products with added sugar.

Why should I pee twice?

Completely emptying the bladder speeds up cure rates and can prevent recurrence. Urine is left in the bladder after peeing (the so-called 'residual volume'), and is like nectar to the bacteria—they feast, feed, and thrive on it.

Double micturition, or peeing twice, is the answer: after voiding urine as usual, stand up and jiggle for 30 seconds, sit down and pee again. If more urine appears at this second sitting, you clearly didn't empty the bladder fully the first time. No more proof is needed.

Bizarre as it sounds, double micturition has relieved many women after years of attacks of cystitis and they continue to 'pee twice' as a way of diminishing the chances of further attacks.

Resources

http://www.bashh.org Enter a postcode to find the nearest clinic in the UK.

http://www.hivtest.org/std_testing.cfm Enter a zip code to find the nearest clinic in the USA.

http://www.netdoctor.co.uk/diseases/facts/cystitis.htm Advice on cystitis.

2

Understanding
your results
Playing with numbers

➔ Key points

◆ Results from hospital tests may be incorrect (wrongly positive or wrongly negative)

◆ Newspaper headlines showing increases (or decreases) in numbers of cases should be viewed with suspicion

◆ 'Equivocal' results simply means that the test needs to be repeated.

In this chapter I shall try to make sense of the numbers we come across when reading, talking about, or being tested for sexually transmitted infections (STIs). I'll explain why the investigations you have at your family doctor or hospital clinic are sometimes unreliable and sometimes downright wrong. I'll explain why the figures for the number of diagnoses of the different infections in 2008 (the most recent full year available) in the UK may be misleading. Before you move rapidly on to the next chapter, saying, 'I can't be doing with maths and sums and numbers', let me give you two examples of what I am trying to explain.

Example 1: in 2008, new HIV diagnoses in heterosexuals who were not drug users numbered 3860 in the UK, but of these only 530 actually caught HIV in the UK. These included 313 with partners who were infected in Africa, leaving 217 infected without risk factors in themselves or their partners. The figure you will have read in your newspaper will have been the 3860, coupled with headlines like: 'Heterosexual HIV infection has overtaken homosexual HIV in the UK', giving the impression that HIV is being transmitted to that extent in the UK. In Chapter 12 you will find out how such a flawed system of reporting coloured our views of the HIV epidemic in the 1980s.

The 1987 AIDS campaign exhorted us not to 'die of ignorance' while at the same time misleading everybody about the extent of heterosexual spread in Great Britain.

Example 2: Mrs BB, a 50-year-old married lady from North London, went to her GP's surgery to have her routine cervical cytology ('smear test'). Because screening for STIs, particularly chlamydia, is so widespread, a test was taken for that. In the interests of 'efficiency and cost-saving', this chlamydia test incorporated a test for gonorrhoea as well. Mrs BB was telephoned the following week by the practice nurse who told her that she had gonorrhoea and should attend for treatment urgently. This lady's husband was undergoing chemotherapy for prostate cancer at the time and this sudden (and faulty) diagnosis of a venereal disease put both under great strain. The gonorrhoea test in Mrs BB's case was a false positive, as it was almost bound to be—see below!

An increasingly large number of persons, whose partner has tested positive for chlamydial infection, turn out themselves to be negative. How is that possible?

Epidemiology

It is common knowledge that chlamydial infection is greatly on the increase— reported cases increased from 59 461 in 1999 to 89 431 in 2003 and 126 882 in 2008. There are reasons why these figures, and others, should be viewed with a certain scepticism (see postscript, page 20). This 'looking at numbers' is called epidemiology, literally the study of epidemics, and measures, amongst other things, *incidence*, the number of new cases of HIV, say, that occur this year and *prevalence*, the total number living with HIV infection each year. The prevalence will include last year's (and all previous years) living cases as well as the new, *incident*, cases from this year.

Surveillance

Why should we count the cases anyway? Well, you must be aware of the spread of infectious diseases before you can control them. If the epidemiologists at the Center for Disease Control (CDC) in Atlanta hadn't been counting doses of pentamidine (see Chapter 12) in 1981, it might have taken years longer for the AIDS epidemic to have been recognized, many more people would have died, and effective treatments would have been long delayed.

Likewise, surveillance detected the new variant of chlamydia in Sweden in 2006 by noticing a huge drop in positive tests (Chapter 5)—the test wasn't working any more! Surveillance watches for changes in numbers and detects early evidence of epidemics, be they food poisoning, this year's 'flu or chlamydial infection.

Sampling

Testing *some* rather than *all* of a population for a disease is called 'sampling'. Not every UK resident is tested for HIV each year, but a sample, those giving blood for instance, is tested regularly and, if the number of positives in this group of people starts to rise, this might point to the start of an epidemic. Any survey is more valuable if the sample can be shown to be 'representative' of the general population. Thus, surveying injecting drug users in the Bronx for rates of HIV infection would not tell you much about levels of positivity amongst married farmers in Rochester. The sample tested would not be representative of all those living in New York State.

Anecdotal evidence

The word *anecdote* takes on a special meaning for epidemiologists. We all know what an anecdote is—it's a story. For the number crunchers, however, anecdote refers to one particular incident. 'My grandfather smoked 60 cigarettes daily for 90 years and died aged 104 when digging his potato patch.' This is just a 'story' until someone tries to draw conclusions, such as 'this shows that smoking is safe' or, less likely, 'digging potato patches is dangerous'. The epidemiologist calls this 'anecdotal evidence'. He would like to see how many people who smoked as heavily lasted 60, let alone 90, years. Well, you say, that's obvious; nobody would be taken in by that, surely?

At the time of the 'don't die of ignorance' campaign in the 1980s, a television advertisement showed a young white woman who said: 'My name is Mandy, I'm aged 22, I've had two sexual partners, and I am HIV-positive. I am not an actress.' When I first saw the ad., I had just given an Italian injecting drug user his negative HIV result. He was very relieved since he had shared needle and syringe on three occasions with a known HIV-positive patient of ours some 6 months earlier. Equally truthfully he could have appeared on television with: 'My name is Giovanni, I shared equipment with an HIV-positive drug user 6 months ago and I'm HIV-negative. I am not an actor.' I am sure that Mandy's story was as true as Giovanni's but the message from these two anecdotes could not be more different.

Ascertainment bias

This epidemiological jargon shows how the *true* number of events, infections, Roman coins, whatever, depends on *how hard you go looking for them*. One year you come across three *denarii* in a field. These are valuable silver coins so you go out and buy a metal detector. Next year, you find 50. You tell your brother-in-law, who brings *his* metal detector and the third year, together you find 200. The numbers have gone up from three to 50 to 200. Does this mean that more coins have been deposited in the field? No, you've just been looking harder.

Once the importance of chlamydial infection was realized and cheaper ways of making the diagnosis became available, it was possible to screen many more women than before. Rather like the Roman coins, the more you look, the more you find. There may genuinely be an increase in the *rate* at which women are catching chlamydial infection (last year it was 1000 a week, this year it is 1200, say), but this will be hidden if you are *testing* that many more. Indeed, this extra screening could even be masking a *decrease* in the number of new infections—nobody can tell. What is certainly true is that publicity campaigns which persuade people to attend clinics for testing will raise the number of reported infections.

When you next read that there has been a 15% or 20% or 30% increase in such and such a sexually transmitted disease (STD), at least pause to reflect on whether this reflects a genuine increase in cases.

Laboratory tests

Whenever investigations are undertaken, be they blood tests, urine tests or examination of samples using a microscope, there exists the possibility that the result is wrong. There may even simply be bad labelling; Mrs X's blood is labelled with Mrs Y's name.

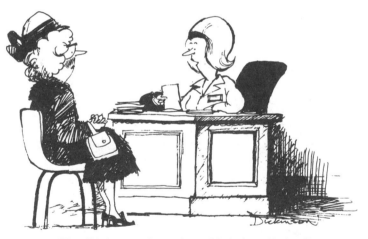

'Why didn't you tell me about this before, Mother?'

Much of the process of testing in laboratories is now automated. One hundred urine samples are set up in a machine that automatically measures the pH (acidity), the amount of protein, the number and type of cells (white or red blood cells, evidence of infection or bleeding), etc. The machine can go wrong or break down.

Today's diagnosis of infection is much different from that of olden days. At the beginning of the twentieth century, gonorrhoea could be seen using the microscope and a diagnosis made in this way was very likely to be correct. It was also possible to grow (the technical term is 'culture') the gonococcus, the bacterium causing gonorrhoea, in the laboratory. Rather like a green-fingered gardener, the successful laboratory technician takes great care with the culture medium, the 'soil' in which growth takes place, and makes sure that all the other factors that influence growth, fertilizer (nutrients), climate (temperature and humidity), environment (oxygen and carbon dioxide content), and so on, are perfect for that particular microorganism.

This sort of 'horticulture' is time-consuming. It takes a good 48 hours for a gonococcus to grow, and is expensive in labour and equipment. However, after those 48 hours it is possible to say 'this is really very likely to be the bacterium that causes gonorrhoea'. Two days or so later we can say 'it is definitely gonorrhoea' and, further, 'it is resistant to the following antibiotics' (the bad news) but 'treatable with these' (the good news).

This sort of test, laboratory culture, has a very high *specificity*. That is to say, if it says *it is* gonorrhoea, gonorrhoea *it is*. Or, of 100 positive gonorrhoea results, all 100 will actually be gonorrhoea.

Assuming the growing conditions are correct, the test will also have a very high *sensitivity*. This means that, if you had 100 people with gonorrhoea, the test will detect all of them.

Sensitivity and specificity

Sensitivity and specificity are central to understanding why today's tests may give the wrong answer, and address two different questions.

The first is: 'If the test is positive, is it truly positive? You say I've got gonorrhoea. Are you sure?' *Specificity* answers the question 'Will there be false positives?'

The second is: 'If I have got gonorrhoea, will your test be positive? Will my condition be picked up by your test?' *Sensitivity* answers the question 'Will there be false negatives?'

I could stand at the entrance to my clinic and tell everybody, yes everybody, that they had gonorrhoea. As a test for gonorrhoea it would be a pretty poor one in that it would generate a large number of false *positives*. But, *and this is of interest*, it would treat every single case of gonorrhoea that came into the clinic. It would not miss any cases. It would be a very sensitive test.

Or, I could stand at the entrance to my clinic and tell everybody that they did not have gonorrhoea. Because almost all the people who attend have *not* got gonorrhoea, this would be quite a specific test. It would be right in almost all the cases. But it would miss the few positives.

The relative importance of sensitivity or specificity can vary considerably in different circumstances. Let's look at examples of how these two concepts might assume different importance:

- **Sensitivity**: I have been unfaithful to my wife. I had sex with a woman without using a condom last week. My wife is returning from abroad shortly and I need to be sure that I won't infect her with gonorrhoea when she gets back. I need a highly sensitive test. If I have caught gonorrhoea, I need it to be diagnosed and treated. A false negative would be disastrous but a false positive wouldn't matter too much since I can live with being unnecessarily treated on this occasion. If the test gave a false negative, I would pass on gonorrhoea to my wife and that would be the end of my marriage. The test for gonorrhoea needs to be *sensitive*.

- **Specificity**: I have been accused of giving gonorrhoea to our au pair girl. Two weekends ago she came home with a boyfriend who spent the night. My wife has forbidden the au pair to have boyfriends to stay but was away that weekend. The au pair has been diagnosed with gonorrhoea and, rather than admit that the boyfriend stayed over, she claims it was me who gave her gonorrhoea. I have not slept with the au pair and I do not have gonorrhoea. A false negative would not matter but a false positive would be a disaster. If a false positive result arrived, my wife would believe the au pair and that would be the end of my marriage. The test for gonorrhoea needs to be *specific*.

Fair enough, so all we need is a test that is sensitive and specific—that shouldn't be too difficult, should it? Well, it is. Problems arise because the sorts of tests we use nowadays do not make use of the old-fashioned 'horticultural' methods of growing gonorrhoea (or chlamydia) which, like planting a cabbage seed, give you a definitive answer. You cannot mistake a cabbage for a carrot, or *E. coli* for the gonococcus. Some of today's tests (nucleic acid amplification tests, NAATs) detect part of the bacterium rather than the whole organism. The tests tend to be highly sensitive—if the infection is there, they will find it. However, this sensitivity is at the expense of specificity. There will be some false positives.

Which numbers affect the usefulness of a test?

We saw earlier how epidemiologists describe, for instance, the number of new cases of gonorrhoea per 100 000 people per year (in London, in women aged 50 it is about *four* cases per 100 000). They also find it useful to describe the number of false positive tests per 100 000 tests. For the test used on Mrs BB (at the beginning of this chapter), there were about *370* false positives per 100 000. Can you see now why any 'positive' from testing Mrs BB for gonorrhoea was virtually certain to be a false positive?

Even though the false positive rate is low, at 0.37%, when it is used to test a population of people who have an even lower prevalence of disease, most of the positives will be false. As screening programmes are further applied, so the number of false positives becomes greater when compared to the true positives.

The NAATs used for chlamydia screening have the same strengths and weaknesses as the gonorrhoea tests. They detect infection if it is present, but also generate a number of false positives. These will, perhaps, be more noticeable when they turn up in an unlikely scenario like Mrs BB's above, but what if Mrs BB had been aged 22 and recently engaged? There would have been no questioning her positive chlamydia result with all its ramifications. One expert from the chlamydia screening programme in the UK recently suggested that the 10% prevalence of chlamydia in young women, a figure generally bandied about to demonstrate the parlous state of affairs, may actually be nearer 5% in the general population.

The 'equivocal' result

Reports from a laboratory that a test is 'equivocal' inevitably result from using investigations that do not culture a particular bacterium (or virus) but instead identify just a part of it.

Many tests use differences in colour with, for instance, a change from transparent to red denoting a positive result. Nobody could mistake transparent for red. A machine is often used to 'read' the colour of a test and its readings might range from 0 (absolutely transparent) to 50 (dark red). So far, no problem. But supposing the test result turns out pink. Well, if it is a dark pink (the machine reads 45), one might say that it is very likely to be a true positive. If, on the other hand, it is barely pink at all (the machine reads 5), most would agree that it's a negative.

What if the result is 25, however? Or 39, or 10, or 16? This is where an *arbitrary* decision must be taken by those making or using the test as to where the cut-off point between negative and positive should lie; and here we have come full circle back to sensitivity and specificity.

- If you choose the cut-off point at, say, 5 (barely pink at all), you will have a very sensitive test—it will pick up the very slightest of infections. But Mrs BB and her husband will not be pleased because of the large number of false positives

If, however, you make the cut-off point 48 (really quite red!), you will have a very specific test—your positives will all be real, genuine, cast-iron positives—but this test will not be sensitive enough to catch all the positives. Some, perhaps early infections, or those in which the number of germs was too few, will actually be positive but the test will not detect them. You will have false negatives.

So how do the decision-makers handle this dilemma? There are two possible solutions.

- The first is to set an (inevitably) arbitrary level, say 25—*all results above 25 are positive and all below are negative*. This approach will give a number of both false positives and false negatives but it shouldn't matter too much since most results will be red or transparent, 50 or zero. And, indeed, it won't matter, unless you happen to be one of those wrongly diagnosed positive or whose infection has been missed

- The second solution is to pick a range of readings, say 15–35 (slightly pink to quite pink), which you term 'equivocal' and on which you postpone a decision until you have repeated the test on a second sample, or done a completely different sort of test.

This has been a necessarily simple explanation of how 'equivocal' results come about. The tests may be compromised by other factors—there are substances found in urine that alter the sensitivity or specificity of an investigation, as may temperature or the time since a sample was taken. If the laboratory is in doubt, it needs to test a further sample. The polite way of asking for a second sample is to call the first result 'equivocal'.

National figures for sexually transmitted infections

In the UK, cases of STIs, including HIV, are collected by the Communicable Disease Surveillance Centre, which is part of the Health Protection Agency (HPA). Scotland returns its own figures and those quoted for the UK include English, Welsh, and Northern Irish cases. As I write, numbers are available to the end of 2008.

The greatest increase, referred to earlier in this chapter, is in reported chlamy-dial infections, which increased from 56 991 in 1999 to 123 018 in 2008. Gonorrhoea increased from 16 798 to 25 410 in 2003 but had fallen back to 16 997 by 2008. There remains a question mark over the chlamydia figures because of *ascertainment bias*, but the other numbers probably reflect reality with reasonable accuracy.

	1999	*2008
Chlamydial infection	59 461	126 882
Gonorrhoea	16 798	16 997
Syphilis	1 118	1 877
Herpes first attack	17 509	28 957
Herpes recurrent attack	14 169	20 361
Warts	71 748	92 525
Warts recurrent attack	39 246	51 682
New HIV diagnoses	2 460	6 377
New AIDS cases	526	505

The total number of new HIV diagnoses in the UK more than doubled between 1999 and 2008, while the new AIDS cases remained more or less steady. This reflects the success of highly active antiretroviral therapy (HAART; Chapter 13). Imported cases, largely from Africa, continue to provide the large majority of the heterosexually acquired cases.

*The figures in this table were taken from the Health Protection Agency's website in July 2010.

While checking the final proofs of this book in January 2011, I discovered that the figures for Chlamydial infection in 2008 on the HPA website had been altered from the 126 882 (see table above) to 217 570. These extra 90 688 cases constitute an increase of 71%.

The HPA's spokesperson told me that this sudden, massive, increase in cases follows from the inclusion of the extra positive chlamydia tests from the UK 'chlamydia screening program'. This extra screening has been running since 2004. But this decision does make comparisons with, say, 1999 (above) somewhat rash, and trends in new infections difficult to describe. Worldwide, epidemiologists' tables and conclusions will have to be re-written. On page 13 of this chapter I wrote (with happy prescience) that "there are reasons why these figures, and others, should be viewed with a certain scepticism."

The second metal detector has indeed unearthed extra *denarii* (page 14).

Resources

http://www.hpa.org.uk UK STD figures.
http://www.cdc.gov/datastatistics USA STD figures.

3

Vaginal discharge and vulval problems

→ Key points

- Vaginal discharge is *not* usually sexually transmitted
- Most causes of unpleasant odour are easily diagnosed and treated
- Water in the vagina has the same bad effect as soap.

The conditions dealt with in this chapter come under the headings of vaginal discharge and vulval problems, the two most frequent reasons for women attending GUM clinics.

A number of genital problems mimic sexually transmitted conditions or may be brought on by intercourse. We frequently see patients who are convinced that they have acquired some frightful condition because of soreness that came on during or soon after sex. This might occur after a period of abstinence and simply reflects pre-existing thrush that was aggravated by the rubbing and friction of sex. There are a number of skin conditions that may make sex uncomfortable or sore.

Vaginal discharge

Every woman tends to be aware of her own 'normal' vaginal discharge and knows that this varies over the menstrual cycle. Others regularly have a little spotting of blood in mid-cycle, coinciding with ovulation.

Is there a normal amount of vaginal discharge?

One might as well ask if there is a normal height for a grown woman. One of the doctors working at St Thomas' in the 1980s, Maggie Godley, asked some of her patients whether they thought their discharge was heavy or light in quantity, or normal. She also recorded *her own* impression of quantity of discharge. She then asked each patient to insert a tampon in the vagina for 1 day. This was brought back to the clinic in a plastic bag and weighed.

What was odd was that there seemed to be no correlation between what the patients thought was a heavy discharge and the weight of the used tampon, nor between that and what the doctor had observed. In short, there seems to be a wide variation in 'normal' vaginal discharge and neither the owner of the vagina nor a professional observer could agree whether there is too much, too little, or just the right amount. Message? Women know their own bodies very well and what may appear normal to an examining doctor or nurse may not be normal for the woman concerned. If you notice an alteration in your discharge, it probably has altered!

There is an expected, and normal, increase in vaginal discharge at puberty and in women taking the oral contraceptive. A decrease in discharge occurs at the menopause.

Should my discharge smell?

No! In the groin there are apocrine glands, as in the armpits, which produce secretions with an odour. This is a normal, healthy, human smell. There are infections of the vagina that are responsible for unpleasant odours, caused by *Trichomonas vaginalis* (TV) and bacterial vaginosis (BV), but neither of them is natural or 'normal'. If there is a fishy smell, then something should be done about it.

Vulvovaginal candidiasis (thrush)

The most common infection found in the vagina, and on the neighbouring skin, is thrush. Probably two-thirds of all adults have candida in their intestines which causes no problems. Candida is excreted at defecation, and both men and women are equally likely to develop infection around the bottom, *perianal* candida. The closeness of the vulva and vagina to the anus makes them liable to infection.

Candida albicans is the most common (80–90%) of several 'candidas' seen in humans, *Candida glabrata* being another.

Why do women get thrush?

The anatomical reasons given above explain the easy route from intestine to vulva or vagina, but there are predisposing factors that increase the likelihood of developing thrush.

- Diabetes
- Higher steroid levels
- Antibiotics
- Decreased immunity.

What are the signs and symptoms?

Candida does not always cause symptoms but, when it does, it makes its presence known in two ways.

* *Vaginal discharge*, described as '*like cottage cheese*', but may be thin and scanty with a yeasty smell

* Candida can provoke an allergic reaction and a small infection can provoke *severe itching*. Occasionally the vulva becomes oedematous (swells up) and sore. The vagina itself does not itch, except at its entrance. The labia, the anus, and the skin between (the perineum) may all be infected.

Tiny, thin, reddish lines (fissures) which are partly sore and partly itchy make the diagnosis of thrush likely. The soreness outside the vagina may give rise to pain on urination, an 'external dysuria'.

🛈 Patient perspective

Mrs SB had intractable vulval itching. This had started a year previously, following three bouts of cystitis treated with antibiotics. The GP took a sample from her vagina (a high vaginal swab, or HVS) to send to the laboratory and prescribed pessaries. Two weeks later, still no better, she was told that the swab test was negative and perhaps it had not been thrush, after all. She was prescribed a weak steroid cream, 1% hydrocortisone, which eased her symptoms for a short time but the itching returned 3 weeks later. During the next 6 months she attended a private clinic four times and on each occasion an HVS was taken and more antifungal vaginal treatment prescribed.

None of this worked and she was desperate when she returned finally to her local practice. When she explained her problems, the GP examined her and, for the first time in nearly 12 months, took a sample from her vulva. This came back from the laboratory showing a good growth of candida species. Three weeks after using antifungal cream her itching and soreness went.

A woman with vulvovaginal thrush may thus have:

* Itching and/or soreness alone
* Discharge alone
* Itching/soreness and discharge
* No symptoms at all.

In men, the itching can be just as intense as in women and primarily affects the glans penis and the foreskin, when present. The glans may become inflamed and raw, with tiny, flat, red marks on it. Occasionally, the foreskin swells. Some men can diagnose thrush in their female partner from the feeling of hotness and itch on the penis within a few seconds of starting intercourse.

What tests might I have?

In most cases vulval itching and vaginal discharge makes the diagnosis obvious. If the symptoms keep recurring or do not seem to respond to the treatment, the diagnosis needs to be confirmed using a microscope or by culturing candida in the laboratory.

What treatments are available?

Two sorts of treatment are available:

- Vaginal pessaries or creams, together with creams or gels for the outside skin
- Oral tablets.

Much drug company money is spent advertising the advantages of one product over another, but it is difficult to show that one product is better than another, and cost and acceptability are the major considerations. Most GUM clinics prescribe pessaries and creams rather than oral tablets, although these are easier to take. Both can be bought direct from a chemist shop.

How should I apply the cream?

Successful treatment depends on eliminating the fungus from the vagina but also, crucially, from the skin of the vulva, *down to the anus*. Fungal infections do not disappear overnight. The cream is used sparingly, twice daily for at least a fortnight, covering the skin from the clitoris to the anus and rubbing it in well.

Antifungal cream can be rubbed on to the end of the penis and foreskin, but any soreness will recur unless the woman is treated.

The combination of antifungal cream combined with a weak steroid may help with bad inflammation but should be used sparingly.

Thrush and sex

Candidal infection can cause problems with sex. A woman with thrush may experience soreness and even pain when having intercourse (dyspareunia), leading to a vicious circle that compromises a happy sex life.

For a woman to enjoy sex, she needs to be in the mood, relaxed, and naturally lubricated. If a woman has experienced discomfort during sex because of thrush, she may well be anxious that it will happen again when next she tries. This nervousness stops relaxation and lubrication, and so the cycle repeats itself. The vicious circle can be broken when the thrush is properly treated and, perhaps, some artificial lubrication is used to help return function to normal.

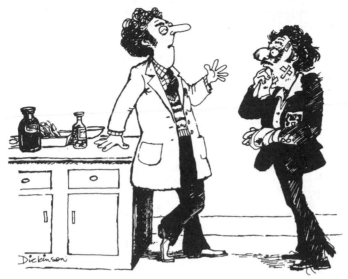

'Your wife is mistaken, Mr Smith. Thrush is not a venereal disease.'

Most women with thrush will be cured following one treatment, but if thrush seems difficult to eradicate it is worth going to the GUM clinic where the staff are used to dealing with this problem.

Bacterial vaginosis

Bacterial vaginosis, 'BV', is a common cause of vaginal discharge and 'fishy' odour and, like thrush, is not sexually transmitted.

Why is acidity important?

In the normal healthy vagina, lactobacilli, the 'good' bacteria, produce lactic acid and hydrogen peroxide. These stop 'bad' bacteria from surviving and reproducing.

The 'bad' germs include *Gardnerella vaginalis* (not to be confused with gonorrhoea) and a hotchpotch of anaerobic bacteria which cause the smell in BV.

The role of some new groups of BV-associated bacteria (BVAB) such as *Atopobium,* remains uncertain. These may turn out to be the microbiological equivalent of angels on pinheads.

What is pH?

You may hear doctors talking about pH, a measure of acidity. Confusingly, a low pH indicates more acid and a high pH less. Neutral, neither acid nor alkaline, measures 7 on the pH scale. The healthy vagina has a pH lower than 4.5. If this reading becomes higher, the lactobacilli stop thriving and there is an opportunity for the other bacteria to replace them and multiply.

So what makes the vagina less acid?

- Soaps, shampoos, and bath gels
- Bath additives
- Douching (washing out the vagina with water).

> Tap water, with a pH of 7, makes the vagina less acid and kills lactobacilli just as efficiently as soap or shampoo.

Many women in the bath open their legs and 'swish' water into the vagina to clean it out. In others water enters the vagina without any help. Either way, you are damaging those vital lactobacilli. It is counter-intuitive but 'the more you wash, the more you smell'.

BV is a condition that only affects women. Some studies have shown the bacteria that cause BV to be present in the male urethra, but there is no evidence that these cause BV in their partner.

What are the symptoms of BV?

Although BV may cause no symptoms, the usual complaints are of vaginal discharge with an unpleasant 'fishy' smell.

The condition is called *vaginosis* because there is no inflammation of the vagina. BV does not cause itching, irritation, or soreness.

Symptoms of BV:

- May be intermittent
- May vary with the menstrual cycle
- May follow sexual intercourse.

This variability can cause problems if BV is absent at the time the woman is examined.

	No symptoms	Discharge	Smell	Itch	Soreness	Dyspareunia	External dysuria
Thrush	30%	Yes	'Yeasty'	Yes	Yes	Yes	Yes
BV	40%	Yes	'Fishy'	No	No	No	No
TV	30%	Yes	'Fishy'	No	Yes	Yes	Yes

What are the tests for BV?

A changed discharge and nasty smell points towards the diagnosis. GUM clinics have various tests:

- The bacteria can be seen using a microscope
- The pH can be measured using special pH paper
- The 'sniff' test.

In the sniff test, vaginal discharge is mixed with alkaline potassium hydroxide, giving a nasty smell owing to aromatic amines with names like '*putrescine*' and '*cadaverine*'. Some women with BV notice the smell after the man has ejaculated in the vagina.

What treatments are there for BV?

Effective antibiotics are available for the treatment of BV, but it is important to avoid the predisposing causes mentioned above. In addition:

- Don't wash your hair in the bath
- Don't douche
- Don't let water into the vagina.

Some women control their BV by putting two cotton wool balls at the entrance to the vagina before getting in the bath.

The main treatment is *metronidazole*, prescribed for 5 or 7 days or given singly in a large dose. A vaginal gel form of metronidazole is available.

Clindamycin is taken for 1 week as 2% vaginal cream or tablets. Both of these antibiotics have a high cure rate. Treating the male partners makes no difference to the cure rate or the risk of recurrence.

Metronidazole reacts unpleasantly with alcohol, which must be avoided while on treatment. Metronidazole is completely safe in pregnancy.

What if my BV keeps coming back?

Metronidazole vaginal gel twice weekly for 4–6 months or oral treatment for 3 days just before and just after menstruation hold some promise. It can be helpful to use condoms for a period to prevent the alkaline ejaculate raising the pH of the vagina.

The addition of bacteria, *Lactobacillus acidophilus*, makes no difference, and live yoghurt may make things worse by infecting the 'good' human lactobacilli with a virus.

Are there any complications of the condition?

Some studies suggest that BV increases the likelihood of premature birth or miscarriage, while other trials have failed to show benefits from treatment.

Yet others suggest a worse outcome with metronidazole treatment. In spite of the uncertainty, the consensus is that it is better to treat BV in pregnancy if there have been previous problems.

The bacteria found in BV may be involved in pelvic inflammatory disease (PID) and metronidazole is often added in treatment of PID or before surgical procedures like termination of pregnancy.

> Vaginal discharge in UK clinics is caused by bacterial vaginosis (55%), thrush (42%), and *Trichomonas vaginalis* (3%).

BV, with the possible exceptions of pregnancy and pelvic infection mentioned above, is a harmless condition.

Common misconceptions

- A vaginal discharge developing after intercourse is due to a sexually transmitted disease. **Not necessarily true**
- It is normal for women's genitals to have a nasty smell. **Not true**
- Frequent genital washing and douching will stop unpleasant genital odours. **Not true**.

Trichomonas vaginalis

Trichomoniasis is a sexually transmitted condition caused by *Trichomonas vaginalis* (TV). It may produce nasty vaginal symptoms in women but often goes unnoticed in infected men.

What are the signs and symptoms of TV?

Like BV, vaginal discharge occurs with an unpleasant smell. Anaerobic bacteria are found along with trichomonads and the pH is alkaline with a loss of lactobacilli.

The vaginal discharge may be profuse and causes soreness. The inflammation can be severe and the vulva may become sore, leading to external dysuria. This should be distinguished from the discomfort found on passing urine in cystitis (bladder infection), which is 'internal'.

Sometimes, the excess discharge leaks on to the upper thighs, giving a sore reddened area known as a 'tide-mark'. Sex can be uncomfortable. However, some women may be infected with TV for years without ever noticing symptoms.

In men, infection with TV can cause a urethritis (Chapter 5), but often it gives no symptoms at all.

How is the diagnosis made?

The distinctive nasty smell and the discharge or inflamed vulva and vagina may give a clue, but a definite diagnosis is made by:

- *Microscopy* reveals characteristic trichomonads moving around
- *Culture* (rarely performed nowadays)
- *Nucleic acid amplification tests (NAATs)* are increasingly being used for TV diagnosis, but there are concerns about their sensitivity and specificity (Chapter 2)
- *Cervical cytology* can indicate infection but (an important 'but') other cells may mimic TV to give a false positive.

TV is found in only 10% of contacts of women with TV, but most are given treatment anyway.

What is the treatment of TV?

Metronidazole is given for 5 or 7 days, or as a single large dose.

In the days before metronidazole, treatment with pessaries made from arsenic compounds was effective but occasionally caused severe inflammation of the vagina. If *Trichomonas vaginalis* becomes resistant to metronidazole, this old-fashioned treatment is a reasonable alternative.

Are there any complications of the condition?

Rarely, a female child can be infected as she passes through the birth canal, and so treatment is advised in pregnancy.

TV (and BV) in the genital tract probably facilitate transmission and acquisition of herpes and HIV infection.

Which other infections cause vaginal discharge?

Both gonorrhoea and chlamydial infection are associated with an increase in vaginal discharge, but neither infection has a characteristic discharge. A primary attack of herpes on the cervix gives a profuse mucopurulent discharge.

Foreign bodies

Foreign bodies are found in the vagina just as they are in men (Chapter 5). The intrauterine contraceptive device (IUCD) is a foreign body (it is *in* the body but not *of* the body) and can lead to discharge in some women. The tampon is another foreign body and one which, if forgotten and left behind, is responsible for a particularly foul, persistent discharge which is, however, easy to treat.

Objects are inserted into orifices by grown-ups as well as children, and foreign bodies turn up unexpectedly as 'aids to masturbation'.

ⓘ Patient perspective

Bridget T, a 14-year-old schoolgirl, put a hairpin into her vagina and couldn't get it out. She ignored it, then forgot about it. Two years later she went to see her GP for family planning advice, prior to sleeping with her boyfriend. She had some discharge and so the GP, before prescribing the pill, took some vaginal swabs and examined her internally.

He was surprised to find two sharp prongs just by the cervix. The hairpin had perforated the vaginal wall, turned through 180° and become lodged. After a minor operation, Miss T started her relationship properly protected against unwanted pregnancy and posing no threat of injury to her unsuspecting boyfriend.

Vulval problems

Itching, discomfort, or pain on the vulva are often caused by candidal infection and the treatment is easy, but there are dermatological causes not helped by standard antifungal treatment.

Skin conditions

Almost any condition that affects the skin elsewhere, from contact dermatitis to psoriasis, can involve the vulva. There are three '**lichens**' that affect the vulva, each different but each helped, at least initially, by strong steroid ointments.

- If one itches, one scratches. Scratching over a long period on a daily (or more usually nightly) basis gives thickened and damaged skin, a condition called **lichen simplex** or neurodermatitis

- **Lichen planus** gives small slightly raised violaceous spots. These usually cause little or no trouble but in some cases the areas of skin become raw and painful, so-called erosions. These also occur in the mouth

- **Lichen sclerosus**, which sometimes runs in families and can affect young children, causes soreness and cracked skin. Lichen sclerosus and lichen planus can both progress to skin cancer when present for a long time, but this is rare and is easily picked up by the skin specialist.

Vulval conditions	Possible causes
Dermatitis	Allergy; irritants; psoriasis
Lichen simplex	Excess scratching
Lichen planus	Unknown
Lichen sclerosus	Autoimmune
Intraepithelial neoplasia (VIN)	HPV; lichen sclerosus
Pain syndromes	Unknown

Cancer of the vulva, like carcinoma of the cervix (Chapter 8), is associated with human papilloma virus (HPV) infection. Vulval intraepithelial neoplasia (VIN) is 'pre-cancerous' in the same way as cervical intraepithelial neoplasia (CIN) on the cervix. Imiquimod has a beneficial effect in the majority.

It is important not to forget the role of 'irritants' in the production of vulval signs and symptoms. Urine, sweat, semen, or faeces can all provoke an irritation, as can sanitary towels, panty liners, or incontinence pads. Some wart treatments, like podophyllin or imiquimod, cause symptoms, and even ordinary soap may be responsible for a nasty reaction. Contact dermatitis, a local allergy, will need a specialist dermatologist to unravel.

With vulval symptoms, *avoid* vulval contact with:

- Soap, shampoo, bubble bath
- 'Feminine' products
- Spermicides (including condoms)
- Tight under-clothes.

What are vulval pain syndromes?

Vulval vestibulitis, provoked vestibulodynia, and dysaesthetic vulvodynia are terms variously used to describe pain in and around the vulva.

Vulvodynia is the 'catch-all' symptom defined by the International Society for the Study of Vulvovaginal Disease, the ISSVD, as chronic discomfort or pain in the vulva which may be 'burning, stinging, irritation or rawness' in the absence of any infectious or skin disease. Generalized vulvodynia involves the entire vulva, including the clitoris and pubic area, or it may affect different areas at different times.

The vestibule is the oval-shaped area of skin between the labia, and between the clitoris and the perineum. Women with the *vulval vestibulitis syndrome* (VVS) have discomfort limited to when, or immediately after, that part of the vulva is touched. Sexual intercourse, insertion of a tampon or a speculum—indeed, anything that exerts pressure on the vestibule—brings on a characteristic burning sensation. Women with VVS not only have their daily routine disrupted—it may be uncomfortable just sitting—but may find it difficult or impossible to have sex. Clinical depression is a not uncommon feature.

Is HPV involved?

Contrary to previous theories, HPV infection is found no more frequently than in the general population. In some women with 'cyclic vulvovaginitis', which comes and goes, often depending on the stage of the menstrual cycle, long-term treatment with oral antifungals has been successful.

How is VVS managed?

Strong steroid ointment, if used for a month or so, gives marked improvement in 30% of women. *Amitriptyline*, an antidepressant, works consistently in most of these chronic vulval conditions, but it is important not to give the impression that the symptoms are simply 'psychological'—these are real physical conditions with a medical, organic basis.

One of the difficulties that arise is sensitization of the vulval skin to all the various products that are applied so regularly. For recurrent candidal infection, it may be better to use oral antifungal agents rather than topical creams or ointments.

A successful, and innovative, approach to vulval pain is the development of a *multidisciplinary team* to look after different aspects of the patient's problem. The doctor, psychotherapist, physiotherapist, and dietician see the sufferer, in that order, and empower the patient by involving her in decisions about the way in which her condition is to be managed.

Many women have only discussed their problem with a GP and few with their partner. The very giving of a diagnosis, the labelling, was found to give significant relief in 85% of women in one study. The recognition that theirs was a genuine condition which carried no stigma put them well on their way to recovery.

The menopause and the vulva

Postmenopausal women may suffer from the unhappily labelled 'senile' atrophy which describes the ageing of the vulval and vaginal skin when there is less oestrogen circulating. Oestrogen promotes storage of glycogen and helps in the maintenance of the healthy vagina's acid pH. Five years after the menopause there is a 30% reduction in skin glycogen. *Atrophic vaginitis* is a relatively easy diagnosis to make which is readily treated with topical oestrogen cream.

Resources

http://www.bashh.org BASHH guidelines on vaginal discharge.
http://www.bashh.org/documents/113/113.pdf BASHH guidelines on vulval conditions.
http://www.bssvd.org/leaflets.asp British Society for the Study of Vulval Disease.
http://www.nva.org National Vulvodynia Association.
http://www.vul-pain.dircon.co.uk Vulval Pain Society (VPS).

4

Gonorrhoea

→ Key points

- You cannot catch gonorrhoea from a lavatory seat
- Many women have no symptoms from an attack of gonorrhoea
- Although most men have a discharge from the penis, only 50% have pain on urination.

Historical aspects

The disease had been recognized by sages such as Hippocrates, Plato, and Aristotle for many centuries before Galen named it gonorrhoea in the second century from the Greek γονη = semen and ρειν = to flow.

The Old Testament, Leviticus, Chapter 15, devotes several verses to what is almost certainly gonorrhoea:

> *when any man has a running issue out of his flesh; because of his issue he is unclean*

with a comment on possible infectious period and personal hygiene:

> *then he shall number to himself seven days for his cleansing, and wash his clothes, and bathe his flesh in running water, and shall be clean*

with even a suggestion that the myth of the lavatory seat as a source of infection pre-dates the invention of the flush toilet by over 2000 years:

> *he that sitteth on anything whereon he sat that hath the issue shall wash his clothes, and bathe himself in water.*

Scientist Albert Neisser is credited with discovering *Neisseria gonorrhoeae* in 1879, but a Professor Hallier had described its characteristic microscopic appearance 7 years earlier. Perhaps it should be called *Hallieria gonorrhoeae*.

What did Hallier and Neisser find?

Gonococci are easy to see using a microscope's high magnification. They are pink (Gram-stain negative) kidney-shaped bacteria inside white cells, arranged in pairs (diplococci). So, the three criteria for a microscopic diagnosis of gonorrhoea are:

- Gram-negative (GN)
- Intracellular (I)
- Diplococci (D).

Very rarely, *Neisseria meningitidis* (the cause of meningitis) gives a urethritis, proctitis, or cervicitis with the same microscopic appearance (GNID) as gonorrhoea. *N. meningitidis* is found normally in many people's throats, and fellatio may explain its presence in the urethra.

How is it caught?

Gonorrhoea is almost exclusively acquired sexually—by penetrative vaginal or rectal intercourse, and oral sex.

How infectious is gonorrhoea?

Nobody knows. A man with gonorrhoea might have a 95% chance of passing it on from one episode of vaginal sex. If the woman has gonorrhoea, the risk to the man will be less.

How soon are you infectious?

Again, nobody knows but there have been anecdotes of transmission within an hour or two of catching gonorrhoea.

How soon after sex can I have tests?

If one wishes to *exclude* gonorrhoea in someone who has been at risk, particularly a woman, it is best to wait for at least 3 days (some say 1 week) to ease detection.

Can I catch gonorrhoea from a lavatory seat?

Well, it is theoretically possible, but it would be extremely difficult. This is because the gonococcus rapidly dies away from the warmth and moisture of a human being. It is just possible (I have never seen or heard of a case in 40 years of practice) that a man's penis could leave a little discharge on the lavatory, when sitting, and that a second man's penis could come into contact with the discharge.

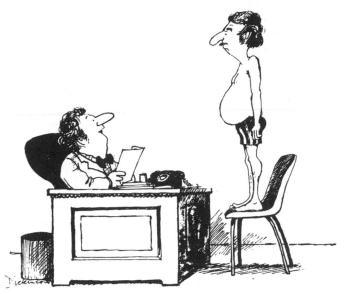

*If I've told you once, I've told you a hundred times.
It's quite safe to sit down!'*

The gonococcus cannot infect ordinary skin surfaces; it needs mucous membrane or internal tissue. It is therefore unlikely that a woman could either infect a lavatory seat or bring an infectable part of her anatomy into contact with one.

A few years ago, a report was published of transmission of gonorrhoea via an inflatable rubber doll. This is rare!

There are two exceptions to sexual transmission of gonorrhoea—newborn infants and pre-pubertal girls.

- If a mother is suffering from gonorrhoea of the cervix when she gives birth, the baby's eyes can become infected, giving rise to the condition ophthalmia neonatorum (see page 53 for chlamydial infection), the commonest cause of childhood blindness in olden times

In 2008, there were 15 cases of ophthalmia neonatorum in the UK

- The eyes, throat, and vulva may become infected, so the baby is given oral antibiotics as well as topical ones for the eye

- The second non-sexual mode of transmission is via inanimate objects such as towels or flannels. Nowadays everyone is much more aware of child sexual abuse and, while this possibility must never be discounted, it does not have to be the case. Before antibiotics, there were reports of outbreaks of gonococcal vulvovaginitis on wards or in dormitories where the serial abuse of 20 or 30 young girls was less likely than the infected, uncleaned, rectal thermometer that had been used consecutively on all the inmates.

❔ Patient perspective

Professor Natalie V., a microbiologist, was transporting equipment to her laboratory while carrying her 18-month-old daughter in the back of the car. The equipment comprised agar plates. Samples are inoculated onto these plates for subsequent laboratory culture.

The professor was horrified to find that her baby had reached over and was quietly munching her way through the jelly-like contents of one of the agar plates from a local STI clinic. Some 48 hours later, there was a positive culture for gonorrhoea in the lab. A throat swab from her daughter also grew gonorrhoea—probably the youngest verified case of oropharyngeal gonorrhoea ever—but innocently acquired.

Can I catch gonorrhoea from kissing?

Mouth-to-mouth transmission between adults is theoretically possible but unlikely. While we often find gonorrhoea in the throats of women or gay men who perform fellatio, it is unusual in men who have had oral sex with an infected *female* partner.

Like infection caught from a lavatory seat, I have never come across a case of direct mouth-to-mouth transmission of gonorrhoea.

Are there many cases today?

The number of cases of gonorrhoea goes up and down like a roller-coaster, with the discovery of new antibiotics since 1950 seemingly having little effect on the epidemic.

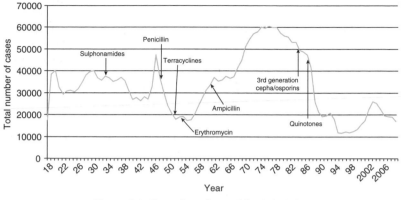

Figure 4.1 Gonorrhoea figures UL: 1918–2008.

Gonorrhoea reached its peak incidence in the mid-1970s, with over 60 000 cases in England, compared with some 11 780 cases in 1994. The decrease has been attributed to changing sexual practices as a result of the fear of AIDS but, in truth, the decline had started several years before the HIV epidemic became apparent. Antibiotics have little effect on the number of cases (see figure 4.1).

Who catches gonorrhoea?

The risk of gonorrhoea is unequal between different ethnic groups and sexual orientations. In the UK, most gonorrhoea amongst men who have sex with men (MSM; over 90%) occurs in the white population while the reverse is true in heterosexual men. Similar findings in the USA show higher rates of infection in those of African American and Hispanic origin.

- Young adults (15–30) have the highest incidence of gonorrhoea (females > males)
- MSM and ethnic minority groups bear a disproportionate burden of disease

Which bits of me are infected?

The usual sites infected are the urethra, throat, and rectum in men, and cervix, urethra, rectum, and throat in women. Rectal gonorrhoea in the male is mostly the result of insertive rectal intercourse, although infection can be passed on by vibrators or digital insertion. In 40% of women with gonorrhoea, the infection is found in the rectum, not necessarily as a result of rectal intercourse; gravity can allow infected secretions to come into contact with anal tissue during intercourse.

In about 5% of cases each, the rectum or urethra will be the only site from which the gonococcus can be identified. So, if one is trying to *exclude* gonorrhoea, it is crucial to sample all sites.

How is gonorrhoea diagnosed?

- *Microscopy* works in over 95% of cases of men with gonococcal discharge. In women, however, less than 50% are microscopy-positive. For all its lowered sensitivity, microscopy does offer the chance of an instant diagnosis in women

- *Culture* (Chapter 2) has more positives than microscopy and also reveals the organism's antibiotic sensitivity

- *Nucleic acid amplification tests (NAATs)* may be prone to a lack of specificity (Chapter 2). However, these tests are highly sensitive—if the gonococcus is present, they'll find it—and they may turn out to have particular value in the throat and rectum

- *Blood tests* for gonorrhoea are discounted—none is at all reliable.

What do men notice?

Discharge in acute gonorrhoea starts as a slight bit of mucus, developing into full-blown pus after a day or two—off-white and staining the underwear.

Clinic workers recognize the 'tissue paper' sign—when a man attends with a piece of tissue paper on the inside of his underwear, the diagnosis is gonorrhoea until proved otherwise.

Dysuria is a classical symptom of gonorrhoea but we rarely see patients complaining of the really severe discomfort mentioned in the old textbooks. These days, half of those attending our clinic in London with gonorrhoea do not mention any discomfort at all.

> Old descriptions included: 'pissing broken glass', 'like razor blades', and 'a red-hot poker in the pipe'.

The other change is the longer time it takes for someone with gonorrhoea to attend a clinic after developing symptoms. In the 1930s the average time was under 3 days, whereas now it is nearer 6 days. Perhaps the pre-war patients were driven by extreme discomfort, lacking today.

How soon will I notice my symptoms?

The incubation period, that time between infection and the development of symptoms, has progressively lengthened since the 1930s. In that pre-war era, men noticed something wrong within 2 or 3 days. By the 1990s, the average time had increased to over 8 days.

One in ten men and half of women have no symptoms from their gonorrhoea

Why has the incubation period lengthened and the pain diminished? These changes perhaps reflect adaptations by the gonococcus to changes in its environment. Once effective and lethal antibiotics arrived, there would be a selective advantage to those strains of the gonococcus that produced *fewer* symptoms, *later*. They would have a greater chance of being passed on to another person before the penicillin destroyed them.

Gonorrhoea of the rectum tends to produce no symptoms in more than 80% of men (or women) infected there. Some notice pus on their faeces and others may complain of a little dampness or itching around the anus, but most are unaware of their infection.

Infection of the throat is not associated with any particular symptoms, although it seems that men or women who practise orogenital sex are more prone to sore throats than others.

What do women notice?

The gonococcus is a microbiological master of male chauvinism, being difficult to diagnose in women under the microscope, and producing few symptoms or signs to lead physician or patient towards the diagnosis.

- There are *no helpful symptoms* at all in perhaps 50% of cases
- Some women mention an *alteration in vaginal discharge* but without particular characteristics. In our study of gonorrhoea, the most common description was 'white'
- *Discomfort on passing urine* is more often caused by UTI rather than gonorrhoea
- The development of symptoms in her partner may be her first clue.

Urethral discharge in a woman is a rare sign, and a rare symptom.

> Cystitis is a more likely cause of dysuria than gonorrhoea in a woman

Other symptoms arise as a result of late complications, like salpingitis.

What are the complications of gonorrhoea?

The complications of gonorrhoea in women are dealt with in some detail in Chapter 6. Local infection of glands around the vulva can cause a **bartholinitis**, painful swelling on the labia, or **skenitis**, a similar condition next to the urethra. Both are rare in the west today.

Spread of infection inwards can give rise to **endometritis**, followed by involvement of the Fallopian tubes, **salpingitis**, and into the pelvis to cause pelvic **peritonitis**. Chlamydial and gonococcal salpingitis share the same signs and symptoms; both infections may be found together in the same patient and both may lead to **ectopic pregnancy**.

Lower abdominal pain (LAP) is a persisting problem with pelvic infection, and is often combined with 'deep dyspareunia', discomfort felt during intercourse. This also occurs sometimes in perfectly healthy women because of contact between the penis and the ovaries. A woman's ovaries are as sensitive as a man's testicles and are normally protected within the bony pelvis; but there are certain occasions during sex when the erect penis will bang the ovary. This is known as the 'anvil syndrome' after the metal block on which a blacksmith fashions a horseshoe.

Spread of infection internally can give rise to the **Fitz-Hugh–Curtis syndrome**, a condition in which the lining outside the liver becomes inflamed, a 'peri-hepatitis'. This is hard to diagnose since pain under the right ribs is difficult to reconcile with an infection originally caught through sex.

Rarely, gonorrhoea spreads via the bloodstream to elsewhere in the body, usually the skin and the joints.

Other 'old-fashioned' complications included hepatitis, meningitis (mimicking its cousin, the meningococcus), and even endocarditis, when the heart valves become infected. The only reports of this condition since World War 2 have come from the USA. It was usually fatal, as a publication from 1938 indicates:

> Gonococcal endocarditis—a report of 12 cases, *with 10 post-mortem examinations* (my italics)

Men are less likely to develop these bloodborne complications but may develop infection of the various glands in the genital area, including Littré's glands inside the urethra and Cowper's, Tyson's, and the prostate gland. The gonococcus also infects the testicles, causing **epididymo-orchitis**.

How is gonorrhoea treated?

In 1937, the *Journal of the American Medical Association* reported the first successful treatment of gonorrhoea using a sulphonamide, M & B 693, to the relief of patients and doctors alike.

Historical snippet

An old treatment was *urethral irrigation*, in which a strong antiseptic solution was run into the urethra under high pressure to 'wash out' the germs. Progression of the infection was monitored by regular 'urethroscopy': a rigid metal tube with telescope attached was passed into the urethra to see how things were going. Ouch!

Penicillin was being developed when gonorrhoea stopped responding to sulphonamides. During the war, penicillin was reserved for soldiers with venereal disease (VD) rather than those with, say gangrene, because the 'VD' patients could be returned to active duty more readily.

Antibiotic resistance

This loss of efficacy of the sulphonamides was the first example of antibiotic resistance.

The susceptibility of *Neisseria gonorrhoeae* to antibiotics differs in different countries, and is related to their misuse. Where antibiotics are available without prescription, the gonococcus develops reduced sensitivity to these agents. *N. gonorrhoeae* is more likely to be resistant to penicillin in the Far East or Africa than in the UK.

A group of antibiotics called the cephalosporins remains effective throughout the world, but there is little in reserve if resistance should develop to these. As I write (mid-2010), there are reports of resistance to the only oral cephalosporin currently used for gonorrhoea.

Is there a connection between gonorrhoea and HIV infection?

Gonorrhoea facilitates *transmission* of HIV and is a good *marker of risk* of HIV. To catch gonorrhoea or HIV, you need to have had unprotected sex. Catching the one denotes immediate risk of the other.

Resources

http://www.iusti.org/regions/Europe/Euro_guideline_GC_2009.pdf European Guidelines on gonorrhoea 2009.

http://www.iusti.org/regions/Europe/Euro_PIL_Gonorrhoea.pdf Gonorrhoea leaflet 2010

5

Non-specific genital infection

Key points

- *Chlamydia trachomatis* is the most common cause of non-gonococcal urethritis (NGU)
- A new bacterium, *Mycoplasma genitalium*, causes up to 20% of NGU
- *Chlamydia trachomatis* causes no symptoms in most women and many men.

Why non-specific?

Non-specific genital infection (NSGI) is a general term for a number of genital conditions affecting men and women, all characterized by the *lack of a precise diagnosis*.

NSU stands for non-specific *urethritis*, an inflammation of the urethra in a man.

Inflammation is the production of white, or 'pus', cells. Pus from a boil is a mixture of bacteria and these white cells.

NSU has a variety of causes but, in many cases, no microorganism is found; i.e. truly *non-specific*.

If the test for chlamydia is positive, the urethritis is no longer 'non-specific' but is '*chlamydial*'.

The most important single cause of non-specific infection, *Chlamydia trachomatis*, is dependent on laboratory diagnosis.

Causes of inflammation in the urethra

- **Bacteria**, including gonorrhoea, chlamydia, and *Mycoplasma genitalium*
- **Viruses**, including herpes and HPV

- Protozoa—trichomonas
- Fungi—candida
- Irritants, including alcohol and hot spices
- Foreign bodies—see below.

The discharge in NSU may be clear to the naked eye (mucoid) or mucus mixed with pus cells (mucopurulent). Pus cells may be present with no obvious discharge at all.

How is NSU diagnosed?

With most infections, there is a test which can confirm the presence of infection. This might be a blood test, or identification of the germ using a microscope or laboratory culture.

In many NSU cases no germ is found

The first indication of NSU will come from symptoms or a history of exposure to infection. If infection or inflammation are to be confirmed or excluded, we need to establish whether there is a *urethritis*; are there pus cells present? This is checked by taking a 'smear' from the urethra, with a small swab, which is examined using a microscope.

'Counting' pus cells

The number of pus cells is counted for 10 different areas (fields) on the slide and is then averaged to arrive at a magic figure, the pus cells per field, which indicates the severity of the urethritis. The pitfalls of such a system are mentioned in Chapter 2 ('Playing with numbers'), and what appears to be a scientific and exact system for evaluating urethritis is nothing of the sort and can result in faulty diagnoses.

Gonorrhoea is effectively the only cause of urethritis that can be *reliably and consistently* confirmed by microscopy.

'NGU' or non-gonococcal urethritis is an alternative label for 'NSU', but most clinicians and patients still refer to the condition as NSU

So, pus cells are found. Does that mean that an infection is present? Well, a heavy drinking session might result in alcohol in the urine, giving a 'chemical' urethritis.

The resulting pus cells look identical to those found with infection. Some suggest that hot spices give a urethritis.

In other cases, where it is inconceivable that a sexually transmitted condition could be present, no explanation for the inflammation can be found.

What are the *possible* causes of NSU?

Since the 1950s a number of different organisms have come and gone as the magical '*organism X*' that causes NSU. I mention two 'possible' causes in a little detail since, in various parts of the world, they are regarded as *definitely* responsible for disease (pathogenic) and are vigorously, and expensively, sought and treated. If either of the two bacteria below have been diagnosed and treated in Milan, Marseille or Mill Spring, Missouri (population, 252), do not panic, just pause before spending any more good money.

In 1971, *Mycoplasma hominis* was eliminated from our list of causes of NSU in the UK. This was, and is, sexually transmitted but is not a sexually transmitted *disease*. In several European countries *M. hominis* is regarded as a pathogen in the urethra but evidence for this is lacking.

M. hominis has been implicated in some cases of acute kidney infection, and possibly in some pelvic infection in women. So it certainly can cause disease—*but not NSU!*

Next to emerge was *Ureaplasma urealyticum*. This little bug earned its credibility when two eminent researchers inoculated their urethras with *U. urealyticum*. Both developed a rip-roaring urethritis that lasted for several weeks and included generalized'flu-like symptoms. It is possible that *U. urealyticum* is, or can be, a pathogen in a small number of cases but, as with *Mycoplasma hominis,* it is so often found in normal folk without infection, that its role in NSU must be a minor one.

Is *Chlamydia* an accepted cause of NSU?

Yes! Several species of the genus *Chlamydia* cause human disease.

- *Chlamydia trachomatis* types A, B, and C cause trachoma, an infectious eye condition; types D to K, the 'oculogenital' types, cause NSU; and various 'L' types cause lymphogranuloma venereum (LGV; Chapter 10)
- *Chlamydia pneumoniae* causes pneumonia
- *Chlamydia psittaci* causes psittacosis ('parrot fancier's lung')
- *Chlamydia abortus* is a very rare cause of miscarriage.

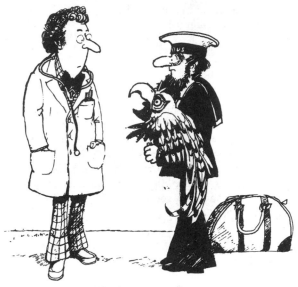

'I caught NSU and he caught psittacosis'.

Chlamydia, as I shall (incorrectly) call it for simplicity's sake, is the most important cause of NSU. Although a bacterium, it lives like a virus—inside a living cell. It can only be grown in cells in the laboratory.

Cell culture is difficult, time-consuming, expensive, and unreliable, and nowadays is confined to research laboratories. Culture demonstrates chlamydia's presence with certainty but, because of its lack of sensitivity (it only grows in 70%), has been replaced by tests that identify bits of chlamydia rather than the whole organism.

ELISA or EIA tests had problems with false positives and have been largely phased out.

Today's tests are variations on nucleic acid amplification tests (NAATs). These have high sensitivity but there is a small problem with specificity (false positives). This becomes a large problem if the tests are used in populations with low prevalence of disease (Chapter 2).

What about false negative tests for chlamydia?

A more worrying recent development was the finding of a completely new variant of chlamydia, nvCT, which had lost the critical part of its nucleic acid used to identify it in commercial tests. This new 'invisible' chlamydia was found throughout Sweden and led to thousands of false negative tests. Currently available chlamydia tests have taken account of this new variant but continued vigilance is vital.

> Several thousand false negative chlamydia tests occurred in Sweden in 2006

Blood tests for chlamydial infection are of limited use in individual patients but may be of use in population studies.

Is *Mycoplasma genitalium* (MG) a cause of NSU?

Yes! First identified in 1989, MG is recognized as an important cause of NSU. It suffers from two important drawbacks. It takes up to 4 weeks to grow in a laboratory and, as I write (2010), tests that are cheap, sensitive, and specific are not widely available.

There is a suggestion that *Mycoplasma genitalium* NSU gives more symptoms than *Chlamydia trachomatis* NSU.

Organisms found in NSU in different studies

Chlamydia trachomatis	10–40%
Mycoplasma genitalium	10–25%
Trichomonas vaginalis	1–20%
Herpes simplex	2–3%
Others	3–4%
No pathogen found	40–60%

Trichomonas vaginalis (TV)

TV is a sexually transmitted protozoon. It undoubtedly causes a urethritis but is only found in about 10% of cases of male sexual partners of women with TV.

> TV is easily visible under the microscope—it paddles around using *flagellae* like oars

All clinics offer treatment to men whose partners have TV whether or not the organism is found.

Candida albicans

Candida sometimes provokes signs that suggest NSU. When this fungus causes inflammation of foreskin and glans, there is often an associated urethritis. This sort of 'NSU' will resolve when the thrush gets better and does *not* need treatment with antibiotics. However, as ever, it is not as simple as that and men may find that they are given antibiotics at the same time as their antifungal cream. Why do doctors prescribe antibiotics in such circumstances? Because people can have thrush *and* chlamydia at the same time and it is considered better (see below) to treat, when in doubt.

Herpes simplex virus (HSV)

HSV is an infrequent cause of recurrent NSU when the ulcers are found inside the urethra. This is a difficult diagnosis to make since men with possible NSU are not routinely tested for herpes.

Foreign bodies

Men and women, boys and girls, little babies even, take pleasure in inserting odd bits and pieces (known as *foreign bodies*) into available holes and orifices.

The vagina is a popular orifice—dildos are harmless foreign bodies—but the urethra and rectum are sites that are fraught with problems when used in this way for sexual gratification. Several years ago a learned surgical journal carried a serious article about the 'vibrating umbilicus syndrome'. This self-limiting condition (the batteries ran down) demonstrated that it is easier to insert a vibrator into the rectum than to get it out.

ⓘ Patient perspective

Freddie P. turned up in the A&E department with pus at the tip of his penis and a burning sensation every time he passed urine. An X-ray showed a radio-opaque object at the base of the penis.

When shown the film, Freddie explained that he had inserted a safety pin into his urethra 'for the purposes of masturbation' with a length of cotton attached to retrieve it more easily. When the cotton broke he had tried to manipulate the safety pin out. Not surprisingly, the pin had sprung open and landed Mr P. in a painful and embarrassing situation that required a surgeon's intervention to sort out.

What are the symptoms of NSU in men?

A major problem associated with NSU is, paradoxically, the *lack* of symptoms. These are often so minor that they overlap with those a normal healthy man might have.

This means that a man with an infection may dismiss the symptoms because they are so slight.

Conversely, and this is more common, a healthy man, because of a genuine infection in the past, may constantly think that the infection has returned and go to his clinic (or clinics) in search of further antibiotic cure.

He may be successful in procuring repeated courses of treatment because of the lack of precision in diagnosing NSU (see above). After a series of such prescriptions, it is not surprising that some men start examining themselves minutely every morning and take the slightest tingle when they pee as a sign of infection. The NSU neurosis has set in.

'Recurrent' NSU occurs in between 10 and 20% of men

Any small textbook or leaflet will tell you that NSU and gonorrhoea share the same two symptoms: *dysuria* and *urethral discharge*. Severe dysuria is rare these days, but NSU gives less discomfort than gonorrhoea. Likewise, the discharge of NSU is usually scanty compared with that found with gonorrhoea—it is rare for the discharge of NSU to stain or mark the underwear.

The difficulty is that this lack of discharge and minimal dysuria may also be all that is found with chlamydial urethritis.

Nobody has yet been able to distinguish between symptoms associated with chlamydia-negative NSU and those found with proven chlamydial urethritis.

So, we have a group of conditions which cause NSU/NGU in men, some of which are *definitely* infectious, like chlamydia, MG and TV; some of which are incidental, like thrush; and some of which are *not* infectious, like alcohol.

The difficulty is that, when the man arrives in the clinic, we cannot tell which is which.

It has been generally accepted that, if a man is diagnosed with NSU, he should arrange that his partner is also treated a) soon and, b) before they have sex again, in case there *is* an infection and he catches it back. However, she may not be too pleased to be asked to attend the clinic, particularly if she feels fine.

What are the symptoms of NSGI in women?

Most women with NSGI have no symptoms, whether or not chlamydia is identified later. There may be an alteration in vaginal discharge but with no distinguishing features characteristic of chlamydia.

There may be visible (to the doctor) changes on the cervix—a mucopurulent discharge and an area of redness. This discharge (likened sometimes to a 'waterfall') raises the possibility of chlamydial infection, but in most cases there is no characteristic 'look' to the cervix.

> Women with uncomplicated non-specific infection are likely to experience no symptoms at all

The inflammation caused by chlamydia in the cervix can result in intermenstrual bleeding (IMB), sometimes following sexual intercourse, although women may bleed between their periods for other reasons.

> Remember that most women with chlamydia do not notice any bleeding and most cases of bleeding are not due to chlamydial infection

Symptoms *not* due to chlamydia

Women may sometimes believe that symptoms caused by another condition are actually due to chlamydia: 'I know I've got chlamydia because of the smell', or, 'as soon as the itching came, I knew he'd been up to his old tricks and given me chlamydia'. In the first case BV had previously occurred at the same time as chlamydia; in the second it had been thrush.

This lack of symptoms, at least until complications have set in, makes chlamydial infection a worry for women. It is sensible to take a chlamydia test at the GP, family planning or GU clinic, whenever there has been a possibility of infection, always remembering that when more tests are done, more false positives result.

How do we manage non-specific infection?

Specialists working in clinics recognize that many people treated for non-specific infections don't need the treatment—men because their 'NSU' is not the infectious sort and women because their partner's 'NSU' is not infectious. Our difficulty is in deciding into which category the men and women fall. Although men in general are less likely to suffer significantly if their NSU is not treated, women run the risk of complications if a genuine infection is there. It is better to over-treat than to under-treat.

Examination of a woman whose partner has NSU, rather than just giving the treatment, may lead to an exact diagnosis. TV and candida are not found as readily in men as in women and, particularly when a man is suffering from repeated, recurrent, attacks of NSU, finding either of these in the female partner can save much time and anxiety.

The diagnosis of NSU using pus cell counts has been referred to earlier in the chapter and there persists a real dilemma in terms of management. For instance, *Chlamydia trachomatis*, an undoubted pathogen, causes a urethritis with the production of pus cells in the majority of cases—but not in all.

So we have the bizarre situation in which somebody with definite inflammation in the urethra may have no infection, while somebody with no signs of urethritis may be infected. No wonder many patients who have had NSU become confused and even neurotic about their condition. Sometimes an attack of NSU can be followed by months, if not years, of needless worry and anxiety simply because, following the mind's focusing on the genitalia, the patient has noticed certain characteristics of his sexual organs for the first time, and normality has become abnormality.

Treatment of NSGI

In the early 1970s, treatment for non-specific infection, with tetracyclines or erythromycin, a macrolide, lasted 2–3 weeks.

Most clinics now use a tetracycline (doxycycline) twice a day for 1 week or the more modern macrolide, azithromycin, taken in one dose. Abstinence from sex is important during treatment to stop reinfection or further transmission before the antibiotics have worked.

Some tetracyclines can make the skin sensitive to sunlight (or sunbeds) and also give a painful oesophagitis if not fully swallowed. Hence the advice on taking treatment comprises three 'S's:

- Sex, No!
- Swallow carefully with food!
- Sunlight, Avoid!

A worrying recent development has been an increasing resistance of *Mycoplasma genitalium* to azithromycin, and longer courses of different antibiotics are needed in such cases.

Does alcohol make a difference?

There have been no scientific trials showing that consumption of alcohol delays the resolution of NSU.

Resource

http://www.bashh.org/guidelines Management of non-gonococcal urethritis—2008 update.

6

Non-specific genital infection—complications

> ## Key points
> - Chlamydia is the most common cause of pelvic infection
> - Infertility does *not* automatically follow chlamydial infection
> - Pelvic infection is over-diagnosed in the UK.

Reactive arthritis

What used to be called Reiter's disease, or Reiter's syndrome, comprises arthritis, conjunctivitis, and urethritis (NSU) and follows sexual intercourse or dysentery. Even after dysentery there is a marked urethritis.

Five infections can cause a reactive arthritis:

- Salmonella (typhoid)
- Shigella (enteric fever)
- Campylobacter (gastroenteritis)
- Yersinia (dysentery and diarrhoea)
- *Chlamydia trachomatis.*

When the condition follows sex it has the sweetly named acronym SARA (for *sexually acquired* reactive arthritis). Possibly half of SARA cases are 'provoked' by chlamydia. Most people with a chlamydia-induced arthritis go first to the rheumatologist, eye doctor, or skin specialist before they see the GU physician.

> An abstinent monk with food poisoning may develop NSU with his reactive arthritis

The urethritis and arthritis can be accompanied by eye problems, thickened skin on the feet, keratoderma blennorrhagica, and shiny red blotches on the glans penis, circinate balanitis.

> Flare-ups of the urethritis in SARA are not infective and do not need
> further antibiotics

The arthritis, eye problems, urethritis, and other symptoms all result from the
immune system mistaking bits of healthy body for chlamydia. Although chlamydia sets the process off, no reinfection is needed to keep it going. Imagine a ball
travelling down an incline. Once the ball has started to move, gravity takes over
and, while it might slow down or speed up depending on the slope, no further
pushing is required.

Not everybody who gets chlamydial infection develops SARA. Of those who do,
60–80% carry a tissue antigen called HLA B27, found in less than 10% in the
general population.

Chlamydia and the eye

The chlamydia that causes NSU also infects the eye. Conjunctivitis follows
contamination by genital secretions and is uncommon. The eyelids are red and
inflamed when pulled back. Eye infection can spread to the middle ear (otitis
media), with temporary hearing loss.

So, chlamydial inclusion conjunctivitis (to give it its full name) needs to be
treated with antibiotics by mouth in addition to local ointments or creams.

> Sexual partners of those with chlamydial eye infection must be investigated
> and treated, however unlikely the link between the eye and the genitals may
> seem

Chlamydial infection in babies

Ophthalmia neonatorum is the Latin name for the 'sticky eye' seen in newborn
babies soon after birth and, in the old days, was due to gonorrhoea acquired
from the mother during delivery. Today gonococcal and chlamydial ophthalmia
have an equal incidence in the UK.

- Gonococcal eye infection comes on a day or two after birth, when mother
  and child are still in hospital
- Chlamydial conjunctivitis may take a week or longer to appear, by which
  time both are probably back at home.

Systemic (by mouth) antibiotic treatment is required because, like adults, the
infection may spread to the ears and lungs.

> There were 39 cases of gonococcal and 40 cases of chlamydial neonatal
> ophthalmia in 2008 in the UK

Complications in women

Confined to the cervix, chlamydia does no harm although it can infect a male partner. Problems arise when the infection spreads internally to the uterus, Fallopian tubes, and other pelvic contents.

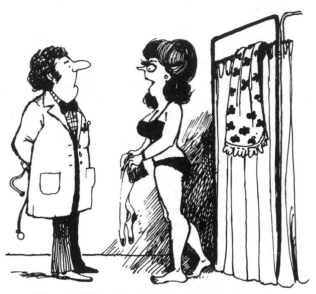

'Not only did my best friend not tell me, it was her boyfriend who gave it me.'

What is pelvic inflammatory disease (PID) or pelvic infection?

Pelvic infection resulting in ectopic pregnancy, infertility, and lifelong pelvic pain is the diagnosis most feared by women attending the GU clinic. *Genuine* pelvic infection actually occurs much less frequently than appears from the reported figures because, as explained in the previous chapter, we over-treat rather than miss cases.

I make a point, as I hand out the advice and antibiotics, of saying 'I am treating you for a *possible* pelvic infection.' We are not sure about the diagnosis at this stage and, in many cases, may never be certain (see below), but it is important to voice this doubt rather than hand down a sentence perceived by the patient as life with hard labour.

In 2008, there were 3834 reports of chlamydial PID in the UK

The label PID includes conditions assumed to be caused by infection that has spread from the cervix to the endometrium, the Fallopian tubes, and the ovaries. When successful conception occurs, the egg is fertilized on its way down the Fallopian tube and has divided several times by the time it implants itself in the endometrium.

What are 'blocked' tubes?

It is more usually *damage* to the tube rather than *blockage* that compromises fertility. Damage to the tube following infection means the egg does not travel at the correct speed towards the womb and either arrives at the wrong stage of development, thwarting implantation, or implants in the wrong place, an 'ectopic' pregnancy.

Acute salpingitis is a serious condition characterized by fever and severe lower abdominal pain. Chlamydia is the most common single cause.

Chronic salpingitis gives a more constant pain, without fever, and may or may not be associated with active infection, although it is usual to give antibiotics to be safe. The pain of salpingitis, acute or chronic, is exacerbated by sexual intercourse, with deep dyspareunia.

Infection can spread from the Fallopian tubes into the pelvic cavity to involve the ovaries. Even after antibiotics have eliminated all traces of infection, 'sticky' inflammation from the fluid or pus can glue the contents of the pelvis with 'adhesions', like a fly tied up in a spider's web. Adhesions can develop over months or even years and themselves cause chronic pelvic pain and deep dyspareunia.

ⓘ Patient perspective

Kylie M. was a 15-year-old schoolgirl with a 19-year-old boyfriend. One Friday, after 8 hours of increasing lower abdominal pain, Kylie was examined at the local A&E department, and sent home with paracetamol and advice to rest. She had told the doctor that her recent periods had been normal and on time.

She returned to the hospital on Saturday evening rather worse, was examined, and again sent home with painkillers. At her third visit on Sunday afternoon a diagnosis of possible pelvic infection was made. She was advised to attend the GUM department on Monday morning to be examined and treated for a possible STI.

It was obvious when Kylie turned up that she was unwell—she could barely walk and was doubled up with pain. When examined, her abdomen was rigid and she cried when it was simply touched by a gentle hand. She had been sick and had not had a bowel movement since Friday.

Kylie was in the surgical operating theatre within 2 hours where her burst appendix was removed and her abdominal cavity, the site of her peritonitis, was mopped out and cleaned.

Kylie's age and her admitted sexual relationship with a young adult had blinded the staff in A&E to a diagnosis which would have been easy for a first year medical student—acute appendicitis.

What are the risks of infertility?

The risks of infertility increase with each infection involving the Fallopian tubes and any delay in treating proven chlamydia. One estimate suggests that 10% are infertile after one diagnosis of tubal PID, 20% after two, and 40% after three.

These figures are certainly too pessimistic since they refer to *proven* episodes of *acute* salpingitis, a diagnosis, as detailed below, that is comparatively rare.

What are the causes of PID?

◆ Chlamydia is an important culprit, along with gonorrhoea. However, between them, these two are found in less than half the cases analysed in the UK

◆ In other countries, gonorrhoea is found in up to 80% and chlamydial infection in 50% of cases. Screening (and treating) young women for chlamydia drastically reduces the incidence of pelvic infection

◆ Some authorities have suggested that the bacteria found in bacterial vaginosis are implicated in PID. For this reason, metronidazole is commonly prescribed in addition to other antibiotics

◆ There is good evidence that *Mycoplasma genitalium*, the most recent cause of NSU, can cause pelvic infection

◆ *Mycoplasma hominis* (the recent, new cause of NSU; see page 47) may be involved in some cases.

What are the symptoms and signs of PID?

Here we run into real difficulty. A clinical diagnosis is made by assessing the *symptoms*, what the patient has noticed, and the *signs*, what the doctor finds on examination. In Chapter 2, when discussing laboratory tests, we looked at the concepts of *sensitivity* and *specificity*. In PID, taking the symptoms and signs to be tests, we find the sensitivity and the specificity (has the patient got PID; is it actually PID?) of both are very low.

This means that, if a patient has PID, they may have *no* signs or symptoms. One expert has suggested that two-thirds of cases of PID are missed because the signs and symptoms are either absent or very slight.

Alternatively, a woman may attend her physician with 'classic' symptoms and/ or signs of pelvic infection yet be suffering from something completely different. This uncertainty is why doctors offer antibiotics if there is the slightest chance that there may be infection in the pelvis.

The textbooks say that vaginal discharge or bleeding, stinging or burning on urination and fever are all symptoms of PID but, at operation, women with these symptoms are found to have *normal Fallopian tubes* as often as infected ones. The same lack of specificity applies to blood tests and other measures of infection.

Why is pain worse after a period?

In some women there is a backwards flow of menstrual blood during the period which, since blood irritates the peritoneum, may cause dysmenorrhoea. This backwards flow could easily carry gonorrhoea or chlamydia. Whatever the explanation, the pain of gonococcal pelvic infection has been shown to come on in many cases at the end of, or immediately following, a period.

If I think I've got PID…?

Women who worry that they may have PID should consult their doctor or go to a clinic, and may be treated as a *possible* case of PID.

It is the practice in GU clinics to see and examine (and usually treat) the sexual partners of women with possible PID and this cycle of events should not be taken, by either partner, as proof of a STI, simply a case of 'better safe than sorry'.

Supposing the pain is in the upper abdomen?

A rare complication of pelvic infection is spread to tissue surrounding the liver, a 'perihepatitis', known as the Fitz-Hugh–Curtis syndrome. It is a diagnosis that is missed because pain in the top right-hand side of the abdomen, over the liver, would not make doctors or patients think of a STI, cholecystitis being more likely.

What else causes pelvic pain?

Probably the most common reason for lower abdominal pain in young women is **endometriosis** involving the lining of the uterus. The blood-rich endometrium grows during each menstrual cycle and normally sheds itself, giving the 'monthly period'.

Sometimes bits of endometrium attach themselves elsewhere in the pelvis, per-haps on the ovaries or lower bowel after the period has finished. These 'satellite' bits of endometrium enlarge, engorge and then shed as the cycle progresses, but in the wrong anatomical site. Excruciating lower abdominal pain ensues, usually related to the menstrual period.

Ovarian cysts, little balloons of fluid on the surface of the ovary, are common and can cause sharp pains when they rupture.

Ectopic pregnancy is a medical emergency. If the fertilized ovum implants outside the uterus, it stimulates whatever tissue it is on to provide blood vessels, just as the placenta grows in normal pregnancy.

This is a literally life-threatening disaster if bowel or Fallopian tubes are involved as massive bleeding can occur. There is acute lower abdominal pain and a real risk of bleeding to death.

What about recurrent pelvic pain?

Many who have had pelvic infection in the past have recurrent bouts of lower abdominal pain over the years. Some doctors assume that they have caught yet another infection and prescribe more antibiotics, year after year. The implication that STIs are recurring, apart from being soul-destroying, does nothing for a faithful relationship. Even the repeatedly negative tests for chlamydia and gonorrhoea do little to reassure women caught in this situation.

The adhesions referred to earlier may be the reason.

What of the future?

You will have gathered that today's diagnosis and management of *possible* PID is unsatisfactory. Researchers have recently found that clinical diagnosis correlates with the diagnosis at laparoscopy even worse than had been thought. Further, it is now realized that there may be infection inside a normal-looking Fallopian tube at laparoscopy. In one series, 12 of 27 women with ectopic pregnancy had normal-looking tubes.

On the positive side, there have been advances in X-ray departments, using modern scanners and newer blood tests looking at special antibodies to chlamydial heat-shock proteins.

What is the treatment of PID?

In the UK it is rare to see acute 'hot' cases of salpingitis in GUM departments. Once a *provisional* diagnosis has been made, antibiotic treatment is started at once and lasts for at least 2 weeks. Tetracyclines or macrolides are the first line of treatment, and metronidazole is often added. Other antibiotics include cephalosporins and quinolones. Whichever drugs are used, rest is recommended, preferably in bed, preferably alone.

Authorities are unsure whether or not an intrauterine contraceptive device should be left *in situ* or removed in women presenting with PID. On the one hand there may be faster healing, on the other, there is a risk of pregnancy.

Complications in men

The epididymis, at the back of the testis, becomes the spermatic cord which leads to the seminal vesicles, where sperm are stored. Infection can spread backwards from the urethra along the spermatic cord until it reaches the epididymis and testis. **Orchitis** is infection or inflammation of the testicle. Most clinicians refer to cases as **epididymo-orchitis**.

Why does age matter?

Under 40, the most common infecting organism is *Chlamydia trachomatis*, or, rarely, the gonococcus.

Over 40, the germs responsible are those associated with urinary tract infections, like *E.coli*.

A man with signs and symptoms of epididymo-orchitis may have either infection. So, as with PID, the man's sexual partner will probably be treated in case of chlamydial infection.

What are the symptoms?

Epididymo-orchitis starts with a dull ache in one testicle which progresses to much greater discomfort and swelling. There is sometimes an associated NSU which may be obvious, with discharge, but more often is only detected on urethral microscopy.

> In patients with immunodeficiency or from high prevalence countries, tuberculosis can be the cause of epididymo-orchitis

A suspensory bandage or 'jock-strap' eases pressure and relieves pain. For years in my clinic the only sizes available were large, extra large, and extra extra large. This at least brought some consolation to the luckless individuals with this painful and worrying condition.

Why doesn't it get better sooner?

I always warn my patients that epididymo-orchitis is likely to last for at least 4 weeks. Patients otherwise expect a dramatic improvement after a fortnight of antibiotics.

> In 2008, there were 1006 diagnoses of chlamydial epididymo-orchitis in the UK

Occasionally a bad attack of epididymo-orchitis affects testicular function and the testicle ends up smaller and softer than before the attack. However, like one Fallopian tube, one testicle is quite enough for normal function and fertility, and hormone levels are unaffected.

What else might it be?

Other swellings of the testicle, with the important exception of torsion, tend not to be tender.

* A **varicocele** is a collection of blood vessels like varicose veins, usually occurs between the ages of 15 and 26, and is of no clinical significance. It is seen more often on the left side

* A **hydrocele** is a cyst filled with fluid attached to the testis or cord which may increase in size quite dramatically ('the man with three balls').

Either of these conditions may produce an ache but not the acute pain of epididymo-orchitis or torsion.

Torsion of the testis is a surgical emergency. Torsion means twisting and this is literally what happens. The testis twists inward by a half-turn or more, blocking return of blood in the veins. The testis and epididymis become engorged with blood and gangrene sets in rapidly. If torsion is not operated upon within 6–8 hours, the testis will be lost.

Who gets torsion of the testis?

The typical patient is a teenager who may have suffered acute pain following an injury during sport. Other cases occur at night with a sudden onset of severe pain. The affected testicle is very tender and usually hangs higher than normal and flatter (the long axis being horizontal rather than vertical). Sometimes similar pain has occurred in the past, suggesting episodes of partial torsion which have righted themselves.

If diagnosed in time, a surgeon can untwist the torsion, secure the testis to stop it torting again, and secure the testis on the other side. If the testis is dead, it is removed because antibodies can develop to the dead tissue which may affect the viable testicle and reduce sperm count and fertility.

Prostatitis

Chlamydia trachomatis is rarely involved in infection or inflammation of the prostate gland. The organisms most commonly isolated are those found in urinary tract infections.

Acute prostatitis gives urinary symptoms similar to cystitis: frequency, urgency, and dysuria. There may be pain in the rectum, perineum, and penis. If bacteria have entered the bloodstream (rare, but it does occur), fever, muscle, and joint pains can occur.

The urinary symptoms can suggest an STI, which is why patients with prostatitis turn up in GUM clinics.

Chronic prostatitis divides into two types:

◆ *Bacterial,* in which causative microorganisms are found

◆ *Abacterial,* also known as 'chronic pelvic pain' syndrome. It is relatively rare to find bacteria in chronic prostatitis. Symptoms include pain at the tip of the penis and rectal, perineal, and scrotal discomfort. Chronic prostatitis should only be diagnosed if the symptoms have been present for at least 6 months. Treatment is with antibiotics and anti-inflammatory drugs.

A brief word about **cancer of the prostate** (which is not associated with chlamydial infection).

There is a heated debate about screening for prostate-specific antigen (PSA), a blood marker raised in prostate cancer. Prostate is the most common cancer in men but:

◆ aggressive treatment of those with a raised PSA is very *unpleasant* for the patient; and

◆ may be *unnecessary* as only some 20% of prostate cancers actually harm the patient.

It is said that a majority of men have evidence of cancer in their prostates, yet die from other causes, having suffered no ill effects. So, we await a good test for early *harmful* prostate cancer. There is a worry that, if more screening tests for PSA are done, there will be more men suffering unnecessarily from the aggressive and debilitating treatment.

Resources

http://www.bashh.org/guidelines Management of epididymo-orchitis 2010.

http://www.bashh.org/guidelines Management of PID 2005.

7

Genital herpes

→ Key points

- *Genital* herpes refers to genital (or anal) infection, *labial* herpes refers to infection of the lips or mouth
- Worldwide, a majority of adults have herpes
- Most people with herpes do not know they have the infection
- Herpes of the lips and mouth is more common than genital herpes.

Genital and labial herpes

'Herpes' is used as shorthand for the two herpes simplex viruses, HSV type 1 and HSV type 2.

HSV1 was classically found around the mouth and lips (confusingly called 'labial' herpes after the Latin for lips, *labia*), and HSV2 predominated in the genital and anal area. Nowadays, *genital* herpes is more often caused by type 1 than type 2 and this is of importance clinically and from a psychological viewpoint.

> By the age of 25, at least 80% of people worldwide have been infected with herpes simplex 1 or 2.

The old-fashioned view of herpes as an incurable, frightful, end-of-your-sex-life 'love' virus has changed. The Herpes Viruses Association, an under-funded and worthy voluntary body in the UK, can take much credit for this alteration in attitude.

How do you catch herpes viruses?

Most people worldwide are infected by type 1 on the face or mouth and most are asymptomatic. Herpes is often caught in early childhood, acquired innocently from a relative with an asymptomatic oral infection. So, herpes is passed on by someone who doesn't know they are infected, and this is *as true for genital herpes as for mouth herpes*.

For 20 years I lectured to 200 or so young qualified doctors on a contraception course in London. The Director, Professor Guillebaud, was always present when I asked, 'Hands up all those of you with herpes?' The great Professor and I put our hands up along with perhaps 12, 6%, of the assembled cream of the medical profession. *Even doctors don't know they've got herpes.*

> Only half of women positive for genital HSV had any symptoms

Blood tests can detect whether an infection has been caught in the past and whether it is type 1 or 2, or both. These tests have problems with sensitivity and specificity (Chapter 2), but can be useful when looking at large populations rather than individuals.

Using these blood tests one can chart how more and more people become infected as they get older and the different degrees in different populations. *Prevalences vary consistently:*

- Women are more likely to be infected than men
- Gay men more than straight
- American more than British
- African more than European
- European more than Indian subcontinent, and so on.

Blood test surveys indicate that fewer young people are infected with HSV1 today than 30 years ago. People who have not been exposed to HSV by the time they become sexually active are at greater risk of genital herpes.

'Genital herpes is transmitted during sexual contact between an infected individual and one who is not infected.' That bald statement brings unhappiness, anger, and resentment, and causes numerous relationships to end precipitately and undeservedly. In most cases not only has there probably been no unfaithfulness, but the perceived 'offender' is the one person with whom a sexual relationship can continue with no further risk of transmission of HSV.

🛈 Patient perspective

Jane and John had shared a flat, a cat, and a mortgage for 5 years. Three years previously, they had split up briefly and both had one other partner, but otherwise had remained sexually and emotionally faithful. One morning Jane woke up feeling itchy on her left labium, but found it rather sore that evening when she peed. The following day it was actually painful when she passed water. By day 3 she found it difficult to sit.

The family doctor was sympathetic, made a tentative diagnosis of genital herpes and suggested she visit her local GUM clinic. Jane was outraged that her 'faithful' partner had given her herpes and attended the local clinic in a vengeful mood.

The nurse practitioner, having asked whether they had oral sex, explained that her partner had been having a symptom-free attack of labial (mouth) herpes, a cold sore, and infected her quite unwittingly. Further, it was most likely to be type 1 HSV, which had a better outlook, in terms of genital recurrences, than type 2.

People do not intentionally infect other people with STDs. Genital herpes is one of the two STIs (the other being genital warts, see *Patient's perspective* Chapter 8) which appear in a faithful relationship. I regularly see patients who still harbour deep resentment for a past partner, imagining that he or she callously passed it on. As far as this common story of mouth-to-genital transmission is concerned, the truth is different.

In the UK, a first attack of genital herpes may result from oral sex with a regular *faithful* partner

What am I likely to notice with an attack of herpes?

In most cases herpes causes no symptoms when it is first acquired. If there are symptoms, itching is followed by a blister or blisters at the site of infection. People feel unwell, with a fever, aches and pains, and swollen, sometimes painful, glands nearby.

The blister(s) burst, leaving shallow painful ulcers which usually heal after 7–10 days. If the sore is open to the air, on the mouth or shaft of the penis, it will crust over and be more uncomfortable than if under the foreskin or inside the vulva where it remains moist.

A primary attack of genital herpes can be a nasty experience, particularly in women. Urine, as it flows over the sores, can cause pain and this was thought to be the reason for some women having difficulty in peeing. We now know that the herpes virus can attack the spinal cord at its lower level (in 'doctor speak', a *transverse myelitis*), interfering with the nerves that control micturition and defecation (pee and poo).

Confusingly, someone who was unknowingly infected in the past with HSV may suddenly develop symptoms for the very first time, maybe years later. This resembles a recurrence rather than a primary attack, that is, not as bad.

Who gets recurrences?

All people who are infected with herpes (remember, that is most of the adults in the world) will have further outbreaks. For those who were symptomatic with their first attack, the recurrence is usually recognized. It occurs on the same part of the body but is not as severe. It may simply be a temporarily itchy area.

The frequency of recurrent attacks varies in different individuals. I recently saw a woman who noticed her first recurrence 7 years after her primary infection. At the other end of the spectrum, the first recurrence may follow seamlessly from the primary attack. What one can say with confidence is that, in general, recurrent attacks become less frequent and less severe as time goes by.

> These days, genital herpes is more often caused by HSV type 1 than HSV type 2

Surprisingly, thrush in women is frequently confused with herpes. In perhaps six or seven out of 10 women who consult me because of 'recurrent genital herpes', the soreness is actually caused by vulval candida. If the symptoms persist for longer than 10 days or seem to be there almost constantly, herpes is less likely to be the correct diagnosis.

Why do recurrences occur?

Nobody knows, but there is agreement on some factors associated with these outbreaks.

- High fever
- Too much ultraviolet light is well known to skiers and sun lovers as a predisposing factor for (usually) oral herpes
- Trauma—some people (this is pretty rare) find that they get recurrences following sex. If these turn out to be real attacks (see above for thrush as an alternative diagnosis), prophylactic antiviral therapy sorts the problem
- Stress—enough people with herpes believe that stress is involved to give it credence as a provoking factor. That there is a psychological element to herpes is undoubted.

How is herpes diagnosed?

The first diagnosis is a clinical one. An experienced specialist will make the diagnosis, having listened to the history and examined the patient. It helps if there is an attack at the time of examination. Coming to the doctor with a typical story, but 3 months after the attack, makes confirmation of the diagnosis difficult.

If an active sore is present, the virus can be cultured or seen using an electron microscope (only available in a few centres). Specific herpes DNA tests may differentiate between HSV1 and HSV2. The DNA tests, like those for gonorrhoea and chlamydia may give false positives and negatives.

Finally, blood tests can tell whether anyone has ever been infected by herpes and whether it is type 1 or type 2, or both. However, unless the infection is really very recent, when a different and transient sort of antibody is found, the blood test cannot tell for how long the infection has been present.

> Blood tests for herpes may give false positive and false negative results

Many clinics, including my own, do not *routinely* offer herpes serology tests, although there are occasions when important decisions can depend on the outcome of serological testing.

> A positive blood test will not tell whether HSV is oral or genital

We saw in Chapter 2 how the prevalence of an infection affects the usefulness of a test. In the general population of the UK, up to 40% of blood positives will be false positives and, even in those attending an STD clinic, that figure will be around 10%. And, of course, there will be a small number of false negatives.

How likely am I to pass on herpes?

Not very, is the simple answer. As we have seen, most people have herpes, a majority with infection of the lips or mouth, almost all of which are type 1. If someone who already has HSV1 is exposed to their sexual partner's herpes virus, as long as that is also type 1, no reinfection will occur. You cannot catch the same virus twice. It is true that there exists a small minority of people who are infected with both HSV1 and HSV2 but they remain just that—a small minority.

Common sense comes into play with regard to when not to have sex. It would be silly to have sexual contact knowing you had an outbreak of herpes, labial or genital.

Some people with genital herpes have entered into long and rewarding relationships with others with HSV, happy in the knowledge that there is no chance of passing herpes on, however often they have unprotected sex.

What is true for HSV is not, unfortunately, true for HIV infection, where the other person's virus may be resistant to all sorts of antiviral agents, and there is a risk that it will replace your own less virulent type.

What is the treatment of genital herpes?

Some 30 years ago **aciclovir** was introduced, revolutionizing the treatment of herpes simplex infections. It had a dramatic effect on symptoms and their duration, although treatment five times a day was difficult.

Because the primary attack is more severe, management differs from that of a recurrence. Aciclovir and its modern variations do not deal with all the problems that accompany a primary attack of genital herpes.

> Women tend to suffer from their symptoms more than men, for anatomical reasons

Acute retention of urine is an uncomfortable semi-emergency. A tube can be inserted into the bladder through the lower abdominal wall (a suprapubic catheter), or up through the urethra, to let the urine out. This can introduce bacteria into the bladder with subsequent cystitis. Avoid if possible!

It is sometimes worth trying to pee in a warm bath, while using an anaesthetic ointment or gel, such as lignocaine (lidocaine).

In the old days, aciclovir use was limited by cost, but when the patent ran out in the 1990s, copies of aciclovir became available at greatly reduced price, allowing for much more widespread use, in particular for *suppressive* therapy.

Also released were new antivirals, valaciclovir and famciclovir. These needed to be taken less frequently than aciclovir but were very expensive compared with the, now affordable, aciclovir copies.

Suppressive therapy is designed to stop recurrences of herpes. It has revolutionized life for the minority troubled by frequent attacks. Given in a more convenient dosage, say 400 mg twice daily, it simply stops recurrences. Some people have taken it for many years without side effects or complications.

Aciclovir as **episodic therapy** is taken immediately any sign of a fresh attack appears. Tablets are taken for 3–4 days only. It doesn't suit everybody but, for those with a reliable warning of an attack, it works well and avoids continuous suppressive therapy.

Once a recurrence has started, aciclovir or other anti-herpes drugs have no significant effect on the severity or length of the attack.

We are often asked if there are medical (as opposed to financial) reasons why we prescribe generic aciclovir rather than the modern, more convenient, alternatives; or if there are disadvantages in not using the new products. Many trials have been performed around the world using these new antivirals, showing a good effect:

- on acute infection;
- on suppressing recurrences; and, most recently,
- on cutting down transmission in couples where one partner is positive and the other is not.

However, the cynics amongst us clinicians wait, so far in vain, for trials comparing the new products with the now out-of-patent aciclovir. We would like to know whether the £80 new tablet is better than the £2 old one.

Topical treatments, creams or ointments, are available over the counter in the UK and are much promoted by their manufacturers. There is little evidence that they alter the course of an attack.

Simply keeping the sores moist with petroleum jelly, Vaseline, suffices for the short duration of most recurrences. The only time topical aciclovir *has* to be used is when the surface of the eye is infected (herpetic keratitis).

> No vaccines against herpes have been shown to be effective and none is licensed for use in the UK

Primary herpes in pregnancy

The main worry about herpes is its effect on the fetus in pregnancy or on the newborn baby. There are major differences between the figures from the US and the UK, with far fewer problems in the UK.

On both sides of the Atlantic there is full agreement about the risk of transmission to the newborn baby if the mother suffers *a primary attack of herpes genitalis during the last few weeks of pregnancy.*

This last sentence emphasizes that the attack needs to be a *primary* (i.e. first ever) attack and that it needs to be in *the last few weeks of pregnancy.* This is risky for the newborn child.

> In the UK, there are fewer than 10 cases of neonatal herpes per year out of 600 000 births. *The risk is tiny.*

Why is a *recurrent* attack not an equivalent risk at childbirth?

Probably the most important factor is the transfer of antibodies from the mother to the baby across the placenta. Along with oxygen and nutrients, the placenta also transmits a ready-made immune package full of antibodies to all the infections the mother has ever suffered from, including this year's common cold, last year's 'flu and, most importantly, her HSV1 or 2. This 'passive' immunity is quite enough to prevent any serious infection taking hold in the baby. Secondly, there are fewer virus particles in a recurrent than a primary attack.

None the less there are some in the medical and nursing profession who perceive a large risk if a recurrence occurs around the time of birth.

> In one large study, HSV was confirmed in fewer than half of 'herpes' lesions found at the time of delivery

There have been several studies, largely from the USA, showing that, even when there are genuine herpetic sores on the vulva at the time of delivery, the baby does not develop infection. Most authorities in the UK agree that caesarean section is *not* necessary under these circumstances.

> In the UK, if a woman has recurrent genital herpes, the risks of her infecting her baby during birth are negligible

HIV and HSV

Those who are HIV-positive and infected with herpes can have attacks that last longer and are less easy to treat and may need to take antiviral treatment in the long term. The best solution, however, is to have the HIV infection controlled with antiretroviral therapy (Chapter 13) when the herpes becomes readily manageable.

> There is no connection between HSV and cancer of the cervix

Some people become emotionally and psychologically involved with their herpes, so that it comes to dominate their lives.

It is easier to come to terms when it is realized that:

- Almost everybody else in the world also has herpes (albeit more of them with labial than genital)
- The chances of passing it on are low and can be even further diminished
- Affordable treatment is readily available to greatly reduce the recurrences
- They caught it from someone who was not aware of their infection at the time and, as likely as not, had not been unfaithful to them.

Resources

http://www.bashh.org/guidelines Management of genital herpes.

http://www.herpes.org.uk Herpes Viruses Association.

Prober CG, Sullender WM, Yasukawa LL *et al.* Low risk of herpes simplex virus infections in neonates exposed to the virus at the time of vaginal delivery to mothers with recurrent genital herpes. N Engl J Med 1987; 316: 240–4.

8

Genital warts

Key points

- There are more than 120 types of human wart virus (human papilloma virus, HPV), half of which cause genital warts
- Most people with HPV infection have no symptoms and have no idea they are infected
- Most HPV cures itself without any medical intervention.

What are genital warts?

Genital warts, properly called *ano*genital warts because they favour the 'back' as well as the 'front', are caused by the human papilloma virus, or HPV.

Warts can occur around the anus in both sexes without anal intercourse

The papilloma viruses infect cells just beneath the skin which, like normal skin cells, move towards the surface, reach the upper layer, die, and slough off, quite unnoticed by anyone.

On occasion, however, the HPV-infected cells form lumps which can be seen and felt—warts. These are *benign* tumours, i.e. they are not cancerous. Just occasionally HPV causes *malignant* changes—cancer of the cervix being the most common.

The most common subtypes, HPV-6 and HPV-11, are found in 95% of genital warts. These, along with HPV-42, -43, and -44, are 'low risk' for cancer of the cervix. There are more than 10 'intermediate' risk HPVs and a number of 'high' risk types, including HPV-16, -18, -31, -33, and -45. I emphasize that only very few genital warts are of the high risk type.

How common are genital warts?

According to one world expert on the wart virus, up to 80% of women will have been infected with genital HPV by the age of 25.

In a funny way this figure, of perhaps four in five sexually active young women, comes as a real relief to that minority who go on to develop actual warts. To know that most of your contemporaries are also infected puts the condition into perspective. To learn also that, by the age of 50, only a small number, less than 5%, still carry the virus tells us that we eradicate it ourselves eventually.

HPV may be less common in young men but will infect well over 50%. Importantly, most of these men and women are unaware of their infection and, unless they develop actual warts, will go to their graves unaffected and oblivious.

So what is all the fuss about? Well, warts are a nuisance. They are unsightly, they don't feel right and it is embarrassing to have them. Certain strains of HPV are also associated with cancerous changes, not only of the cervix in women but less commonly of the penis, anus, and rectum.

How do you catch warts?

Genital warts are sexually transmitted. Most HPV infections give no symptoms so, like other STIs, transmission occurs unwittingly.

> You cannot catch genital warts from towels, flannels, or sheets

ⓘ Patient perspective

Mrs Beryl C. was 35 when she became pregnant. She and her husband of 8 years had both had previous sexual relationships. At her first antenatal visit she mentioned 'bumps' on her labia which first appeared at about 12 weeks. The nurse told her that she had genital warts, that they were sexually transmitted, and that she should attend the local GUM clinic.

When I saw her she was very upset, having accused her husband of being unfaithful (he had strongly denied an affair; she hadn't believed him), and was determined to terminate the pregnancy, not wanting to bring a child into a faltering relationship.

When I explained the figures for asymptomatic infection, told her that many of her colleagues were probably infected, and she might have been infected for 10 or 15 years, she was somewhat mollified but was still suspicious about the sudden appearance of her warts. An explanation that in pregnancy the immune system becomes less aggressive so as not to harm the unborn child, allowing warts to surface, eventually put her mind at rest.

Those who know they've had warts in the past and those with latent HPV infection may develop warts when they become pregnant. The good news is that the warts tend to regress, even without treatment, after the baby is born. Mrs BC insisted that her spouse attend the clinic and, with her newfound knowledge, was not too surprised that he turned out to have no evidence of warts at all.

Genital warts may appear for the first time in pregnancy

The anogenital HPV types are usually confined to the nether regions. Rarely, a mother with genital infection can pass this on during birth, leading to laryngeal warts in her child.

What do they look like?

Not all warts look the same.

- They can be flat or raised above the surrounding skin. In a moist area, they have a softer surface and are known as **exophytic warts**
- On skin exposed to the air, the wart has a harder, 'keratinized', surface. These are known as **sessile or papular warts**. Warts can be as small as a pinhead or as large as a sprout.

All sorts of lumps or bumps in the genital area get mistaken for warts and there are six other diagnoses that regularly cause confusion.

How easy is it to get the diagnosis right?

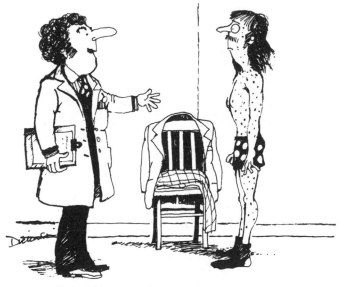

'Relax! It's not syphilis, you've got smallpox.'

'Warts' that aren't warts

1) **Sebaceous cysts** are pockets of secretion from sebaceous glands in the skin and occur almost anywhere. They vary in size from a small ballbearing to a billiard ball or larger

2) **Folliculitis** is, literally, an inflammation of a hair follicle. Any bit of skin that has hair follicles can develop folliculitis which, when infected, becomes a boil

3) **Molluscum contagiosum** (Chapter 11) is sometimes mistaken for HPV infection

4) **Skin tags** are little extra bits of skin near the entrance to the vagina or around the anus

5) **Fordyce tubercles** or 'pearly papules' appear as a ring of small, whitish bumps less than a millimetre across, encircling the glans penis just where it joins the shaft. They are *normal* variations but are often misdiagnosed as warts

6) **Vulval papillosis**, a woman's equivalent to Fordyce tubercles, are little fleshy bumps, also smaller than 1 mm across, on the inside of the labia.

Both vulval papillosis and Fordyce tubercles will not go away if subjected to anti-wart treatment!

Any condition that can cause lumps or bumps on the skin will be confused with warts. However, the six conditions described above will account for 95% of the 'warts' that turn out not to be warts.

Are there other ways of diagnosing warts/HPV infection?

A 'clinical' diagnosis by an experienced nurse or doctor suffices in most cases. Occasionally the changes in the skin of the penis or vulva are minor and difficult to see; some practitioners advocate applying 5% acetic acid which is said to give a whitish appearance when HPV is present.

Taking a sample of the wart (biopsy) and then examining it under the microscope (histology) can give an accurate diagnosis when needed, and identification of the HPV DNA (not available routinely) is a specific and sensitive means of diagnosis.

How can I get rid of my warts?

When we see wart infections in a GU clinic, what we offer is a 'cosmetic' solution. This means we do our best to eliminate visible warts, but we cannot *eradicate* HPV.

So, two important messages to grasp:

 - We can get rid of the troublesome lumps, in most cases fairly rapidly
 - The virus infection will go, without outside intervention, as time goes by.

How do we get rid of these visible warts?

Electrocautery uses a metal prong which literally burns the wart away. It cannot distinguish between wart and normal flesh, so a steady hand is needed. As in a busy restaurant kitchen, an extractor fan helps to disperse the fumes. Not many units still use this method.

The **carbon dioxide laser** is useful when there are many warts, but the equipment is expensive and the 'fumes' given off during the procedure may contain potentially infectious wart virus DNA.

Cryotherapy is the most commonly used treatment in clinics. A jet of liquid nitrogen freezes the wart until it turns white. This is repeated at weekly intervals until the warts are gone. Freezing destroys the skin cell in which the virus resides. The cell dies, the virus dies.

There are two theories to freezing warts. One freezes the wart and a small area around it, whereas the other limits the white (frozen) area to the wart. There is no good evidence that either works better and, since freezing non-warty skin is painful, I concentrate on the wart alone.

Trichloroacetic acid (TCA), like electrocautery, burns away the wart. Care is needed not to damage normal skin and leave scars.

Podophyllin, a plant extract, stops cells dividing, which means that the virus dies out. Podophyllin has been replaced by podophyllotoxin.

Some clinicians suggest that, if podophyllin and cryotherapy are used together, the warts go more quickly than when only one is used.

> All products containing podophyllin are contraindicated in pregnancy

5-fluorocytosine is useful for warts that are difficult to reach, for instance inside the urethra in the male.

Home treatments

Two treatments, both of which can be used at home, have eased the burden for those whose warts do not disappear quickly or readily.

- The first home treatment is **podophyllotoxin,** easy for the patient to apply as a cream or a lotion. Used three times weekly, for 4 weeks, a mirror is supplied for those difficult sites

- **Imiquimod,** an immune modulator, is applied, like podophyllotoxin, three times per week for 4 weeks (it can be used for as long as 16 weeks). Imiquimod and podophyllin are contraindicated in pregnancy.

Both of these can cause soreness, particularly if spread on normal uninfected skin, so care is needed.

What about rectal warts?

Proctoscopy, passing a metal cylinder through the anus to get at the warts, was a regular and standard procedure to treat internal warts. Most doctors now acknowledge that not only is this uncomfortable for the recipient but that *it makes very little difference* to the final outcome.

These days many clinics treat internally only if there is bleeding or the warts are very large. Surgery, particularly if warts are just inside the anus or rectum, may help, but there is a high chance of recurrence within a few months.

Why won't my warts go away?

It is not possible to predict how long treatment will be needed. In some, two or three 'shots' of cryotherapy suffices, while in others the wretched warts just go on and on and on and on. A poor immune system following liver or kidney transplant, or pregnancy, is an easy explanation but for most the outcome seems random and inexplicable. However, in this particular lottery everyone is a winner—warts always go eventually.

It is important not to lose too much sleep over genital warts and particularly important not to let them become the object of an obsession. If the warts are less than 1 millimetre in diameter or so small that a magnifying glass is needed to demonstrate them, *they can be ignored*! Once you remember that they will go away of their own accord and that most sexually active contemporaries will already be infected with HPV, relax and worry about something else.

* At least 80% of sexually active women will have been infected by HPV at some time
* Less than 5% of women aged 50 or more are still infected with HPV

Vaccines against HPV

In the past 5 years, two vaccines have been shown to stop HPV infection, and it is now public policy, in countries which can afford it, to vaccinate all young girls against HPV before they become sexually active.

Tomorrow's generation of women may miss out on the tedium of regular smear tests, never suffer from genital warts and, most importantly of all, be largely free from cervical cancer.

There is quite a case to be made for vaccinating boys since they pass on HPV to women as well as having warts themselves.

Although the two HPV vaccines were primarily designed to reduce the risk of cervical cancer in women, they also reduce the likelihood of genital warts in general and have some effect even on those already infected.

Cancer of the cervix

Up to 50% of sexually active women develop HPV infection on their cervix. Infection persists in 10%, of whom half may develop abnormalities. Perhaps one in five of those with abnormalities will need further treatment to prevent development of cancer.

Risk factors for cervical cancer

* Early sexual intercourse
* Multiple sexual partners
* The socially disadvantaged
* Many STIs
* Smoking
* (Slight extra risk in those on oral contraceptives).

Why don't I have a smear test when I am 17?

The screening system of cervical smear tests has been one of the most successful public health measures over the past 30 years, and has radically reduced the number of cases of cervical cancer. However, there are pitfalls if the tests are performed on very young women.

Smear tests of those under 20 often show suspicious looking findings which *do not mean early cancerous changes*. However, proper investigation can damage the cervix. Most clinicians believe it is better *not* to perform cervical cytology until women are at least 21. Some suggest waiting until 25.

New tests combining cytology with HPV identification will, when generally available, further cut down the need for regular smear tests.

Colposcopy enables the operator to examine the surface of the cervix under magnification. Biopsies can be taken and, if the laboratory shows suspicious cells, it is a simple matter to remove the offending tissue by freezing, burning or cutting off, or a combination of these.

Resources

http://www.bashh.org/guidelines Management of genital warts in UK.

http://www.cdc.gov/std/hpv/stdfact-hpv Management of genital warts in USA.

http://www.cancerhelp.org.uk/about-cancer/.../what-is-the-hpv-virus Cancer of the cervix.

9

Syphilis and related diseases

➡ Key points

- The sore in syphilis is usually painless
- The rash in syphilis is not usually itchy
- Many patients with syphilis have never had symptoms.

Historical aspects

There are two views as to the origin of syphilis in Europe: some blame Columbus (actually probably his crew) for bringing syphilis to Barcelona from North America in 1493. The siege of Naples took place the following year when some, presumably infected, Spaniards joined Charles VIII of France as mercenaries. By the spring of 1495 such a dreadful plague had broken out amongst those involved that the siege collapsed and a disorganized retreat ensued.

The fleeing mercenaries tended to blame the disease on 'damned foreigners'.

The English called it the French disease; the French the Italian disease; the indecisive Italians called it the French disease *and* the Spanish disease; while the Spanish called it the disease of Hispaniola.

The French aggressors were eventually blamed and syphilis became known as the '*morbus gallicus*', the Latin for French disease.

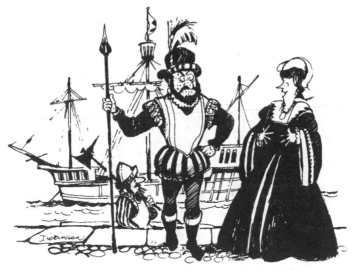

'What have you brought me back from the New World this time?'

The 'pre-Columbian' school argues that syphilis was around in Europe in pre-Christian days.

There are many references in the Old Testament to conditions with signs and symptoms that would do well for syphilis.

One translation, from Psalms, threatens '… the Lord shall smite you in the knees, and in the legs, with a sore botch that cannot be healed from the sole of thy foot to the top of thy head'. Ouch!

Are there many cases today?

Syphilis in the UK, like gonorrhoea, peaked at the end of World War 2, after which the number dropped precipitously up to the mid-1950s. It remained rare until almost the end of the twentieth century, and was largely confined to homosexual men.

The majority of syphilis cases (76%) had anonymous sexual partners

Over the past 10 years there have been outbreaks of syphilis amongst heterosexuals in the UK, associated with commercial sex work and crack cocaine use.

Being treated for syphilis does not make you immune. You can catch syphilis more than once

The chart shows the increase in the number of cases in the 10 years from 1999.

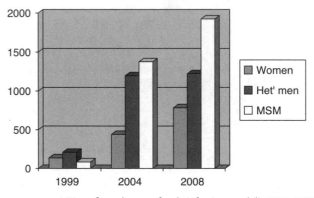

UK confirmed cases of early infectious syphilis 1999–2008

Disturbingly, more than 50% of men who have sex with men (MSM) with syphilis are also HIV-positive. The epidemic is taking place in an increasing culture of unsafe sex, particularly with partners whose HIV status is unknown. Internet chat rooms add to the 'traditional' venues such as saunas, clubs, and cruising grounds.

The social and political changes in the old USSR brought about a volcanic increase in cases of syphilis in the early 1990s. This epidemic headed towards

In 2008 MSM accounted for 61% of infectious syphilis male cases

the Baltic States and was largely found among injecting drug users and heterosexuals, although infections amongst MSM are now increasing.

What causes syphilis?

Syphilis is caused by *Treponema pallidum*, a thin, spiral, flexible bacterium. It invades any part of the body and, before antibiotics, people suffered from syphilis of the nervous system, heart, and blood vessels. The treponeme needs a small cut or abrasion in the skin to cause infection, perhaps one of the reasons it is common amongst MSM, since anal intercourse is more traumatic than vaginal sex.

Syphilis is readily passed on by oral sex, fellatio and cunnilingus

Acquired syphilis is almost invariably the result of sexual activity, while *congenital* syphilis is transmitted to the developing fetus *in utero*.

How is it diagnosed?

Dark-ground or dark-field microscope examination looks at a little fluid from the primary sore or the secondary rash. This test is not easy and is not always successful.

Serological tests for syphilis (STS) measure the presence of antibodies to syphilis in the blood. There are two distinct varieties of tests.

◆ **Treponemal** antibody tests, such as the TPHA, TPPA, FTA or EIA, stay positive *forever* even after successful treatment. These continuing positive simply say that the person has had the infection *in the past*

◆ **Non-treponemal** antibody tests, such as the VDRL and the RPR tell us whether the syphilis is still *active,* depending on how strongly positive the test is. This distinguishes between a positive treponemal test owing to old treated infection or a new infection.

There is a risk of false positive and false negative results (Chapter 2). A positive STS should be repeated before starting treatment.

Modern 'point-of-care' STS combine both types of test and can be used for an 'instant' diagnosis.

What are the symptoms and stages of acquired syphilis?

A sore, the *primary chancre,* characterizes the **first stage of syphilis** and appears up to 12 weeks after infection. Treatment of the sore with antiseptics or antibiotic creams has no effect since the treponeme has already infected the nearby lymph nodes. The sore is usually painless (as are the swollen nearby lymph glands) and feels like a small hard button just below the skin surface. It varies between barely visible to the size of a small fingernail.

The chancre is hard to miss when found on the penis but difficult when on the vulva, vagina, or cervix; or in either sex when near the anus. A chancre can be found on the lips, nipples, tongue, or other sites. One unlucky site is the base of the penis, a 'condom chancre', when a sore on the vulva has come into contact with the lower part of the penis not covered by the condom.

The primary sore is still present in perhaps 15% of secondary stage cases

By the time **the secondary stage** has started, some 6–8 weeks after the primary sore, the bacterium has spread throughout the body. It might seem that the skin rash, which occurs in three-quarters of people, is the most important problem. However, the treponeme can be found affecting all the parts of the body, from the liver to the lungs and the brain to the bones. People with secondary syphilis feel generally unwell, with a temperature, aches and pains, and loss of appetite. Half of them have enlarged lymph glands.

There is involvement of the central nervous system in perhaps 20% of cases of secondary syphilis, with nothing more than a slight headache to show for it. The eyes, liver, joints, and bones can be involved but will all be difficult to diagnose without the coincidental and helpful skin and mucous membrane signs.

After some weeks the rash and other complications of secondary syphilis disappear and the disease enters its **early latent** stage, lasting for 2 years without signs or symptoms although infectious bacteria are still present in the tissues. Rarely, the rash or other complications return for a short while.

In some cases that have been treated, relapse of infection occurs and it is for this reason that patients are followed up for 2 years following treatment. It should be said that when syphilis reappears reinfection is rather more common than relapse.

Active syphilis in the first 2 years after treatment may be a *relapse* or a *reinfection*

The **late latent stage** heralds a period with virtually no chance of syphilis being passed on. Many who have reached this stage can look forward to no further trouble from their infection and will die of old age or an unrelated condition. Those in whom syphilis does continue to be active, progress to **late** syphilis.

The lesion in **tertiary syphilis** is known as the gumma. A gumma results from blockage of small arteries and can cause spots and lumps or nodules in skin, tongue, bones, muscles, and internal organs. These later manifestations of syphilis are very, very uncommon in the western world today.

In the UK, heterosexual men and women with syphilis are increasingly of white ethnicity—63% in 2008 compared with 27% in 1999

Cardiovascular syphilis—10% of patients with untreated syphilis develop disease of the heart and major blood vessels. There are three important complications:

- **Aortic regurgitation**, where the aortic valve becomes 'leaky', putting a huge strain on the heart muscle

- **Coronary ostial stenosis** narrows the opening of the coronary arteries, leading to angina or a heart attack

- **Aneurysms** are swellings in the wall of the aorta or other major blood vessels.

Neurosyphilis is involvement of the nervous system.

- In **general paralysis of the insane**, or **GPI**, there is progressive deterioration in brain function, often noticed only by close friends or relatives but not by the person themself. The memory is lost and judgement is impaired. This classically progresses to delusions of grandeur. The gradually increasing dementia is accompanied by physical decline

- **Tabes dorsalis** involves the spinal cord rather than the brain, leading to numbness and 'tingling', an inability to balance when the eyes are shut, and sharp, shooting, 'lightning pains' in the lower limbs. Bowel and bladder function are disturbed, along with sexual anaesthesia in women and impotence in men. Minor damage to joints is not noticed and severe arthritis eventually develops. Optic atrophy leading to blindness occurs in 20%.

Congenital syphilis

Syphilis can be passed on to the unborn fetus if the mother is infected. The father cannot directly infect the fetus without first infecting the mother. The longer the mother has had syphilis, the lower the risk of it being passed on and the less severe will be the congenital syphilis if it *is* passed on. Thus a woman with early infectious syphilis will either miscarry or give birth to a stillborn child. If the mother has early latent syphilis there is a 20% chance that the child will be unaffected, rising to 70% unaffected in late syphilis.

A pregnant woman's blood is tested for syphilis in most countries, which explains why congenital syphilis is comparatively rare.

In the UK fewer than 20 cases of congenital syphilis occur each year

However, an estimated 1 million children are born with congenital syphilis each year worldwide, and 10% of pregnant women in Africa are said to be infected with syphilis.

Congenital syphilis is classified as *early* or *late*, with the dividing line at 2 years of age. There is no primary stage in congenital syphilis.

The affected baby may be quite normal at birth or may have the neonatal equivalent of the secondary stage with rash and enlarged lymph nodes. The mucous membrane lesions lead to 'snuffles' with a nasal discharge, classically 'teeming' with treponemes. This is highly infectious to anyone who comes into contact, apart from the mother who cannot catch it again because she already has the disease.

The most common manifestation of *late* congenital syphilis is interstitial keratitis, a clouding of the cornea in front of the eye. Late neurological complications can occur, but cardiovascular complications are virtually never seen.

Evidence of early infection may persist in the form of scars and deformities, including abnormalities such as Hutchinson's teeth. If the nasal infection was severe, there is a characteristic facial appearance, a typical 'bulldog' appearance. However, many with congenital syphilis have only abnormal blood tests to show for their infection.

What is the treatment?

The treponeme is sensitive to a variety of antibiotics, but before penicillin was discovered in the 1930s, a succession of treatments appeared to work simply because the signs and symptoms of early infectious syphilis, the chancre and rash, get better of their own accord in a short time.

Evolution of treatment

14th century	Ointment of delphinium, gum-resin, lead oxide, old pig's fat, and mercury which caused the teeth to fall out and belly ache
16th century	Poet Von Hutten promotes a new cure, guaiacum, convincing until Von Hutten himself dies of syphilis aged 35
18th century	Thomas Dover advocates metallic mercury instead of mercury compounds—fewer side effects
20th century	Arsenic (salvarsan), bismuth injections, malaria, followed by heating patient to a high temperature (fever box therapy)

What is the modern treatment of syphilis?

Penicillin has remained the mainstay of management. The treponeme shows no sign of developing resistance to penicillin or any other antibiotics. Daily injections have been replaced by long-acting forms of penicillin, given weekly, although benzathine penicillin, the longer lasting form, may be less good at treating neurosyphilis. Other antibiotics, including tetracyclines and macrolides, are used when there is penicillin allergy.

The *Jarisch–Herxheimer* reaction, usually shortened to the 'Herxheimer' reaction, is a side effect that occurs with treatment for syphilis. The dying treponemes release inflammatory substances and cause a 'flu-like illness lasting 12–24 hours with headache, aches and pains in muscles and joints, and fever. It occurs most frequently, and least dangerously, in perhaps 50% of early syphilis treatments. In late syphilis it is rare but, when it occurs, can have catastrophic results. A Herxheimer reaction involving the opening to the coronary arteries can cause a heart attack. I have seen a patient develop paralysis of both legs owing to blockage of the small arteries supplying the spinal cord following his first penicillin injection. Luckily in this case full function returned within 3 days. Anti-inflammatory drugs such as steroids may be given in the hope of preventing such occurrences.

Do syphilis and HIV infection interact?

We do not know why HIV-positive persons are over-represented amongst gay men with syphilis. It may be that both infections are found with unsafe sexual practices or because active syphilis makes HIV transmission more likely; or

In one report 30–40% of MSM with syphilis were HIV-positive in Brighton and Amsterdam, 50% in Paris and Berlin, and 60% in London

perhaps having HIV makes the transmission of *syphilis* more likely.

Does HIV infection alter syphilis?

The primary chancre is usually (in two-thirds of cases) a *single* ulcer; whereas in HIV infection two-thirds have *multiple* ulcers. It also seems that the primary chancre remains present in the secondary stage more frequently (at 45%, three times more often). Anecdotes (Chapter 2) suggest that involvement of the nervous system may be more common and the disease in general progresses more rapidly.

There have also been stories of secondary syphilis patients with totally negative blood tests. More data are needed. There are few studies, or even anecdotes, about *late* syphilis in HIV-positive individuals. The standard treatment, in amount and length, seems to work with equal efficiency irrespective of HIV status.

Tropical treponematoses

There are four conditions caused by bacteria virtually identical to *Treponema pallidum* which cause problems because their blood test results are identical to those found in syphilis.

- **Yaws** used to be endemic in parts of Africa, South America, Indonesia, Australia, and the West Indies. The bacterium in yaws is called *Treponema pertenue* but it is not sexually transmitted and is usually acquired in early childhood by innocent contact with another infected child. The 'primary' sore, known as the 'mother yaw', often occurs on the leg and, like the chancre in syphilis, is painless. It is often impossible, when assessing someone from an endemic area who has positive STS, to know whether these are due to yaws or syphilis, so it is customary to treat with an 'insurance' injection of penicillin.

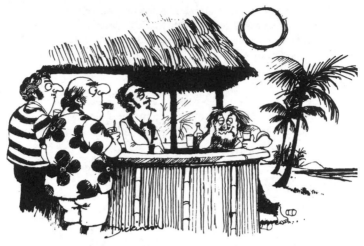

'Tragic! Brilliant physician, but patients kept asking him "What's Yaws, Doc?"'

- **Bejel,** known as *loath* and *firzal* in the Middle East and *dichuchwa* in Botswana, can also present with skin and mucous membrane lesions. Like yaws, most infections occur in childhood, and it is said that adults who have escaped infection when young can be infected by their own children, a reversal of roles from congenital syphilis. As with yaws, penicillin is the treatment of choice.

- **Pinta,** found in Central and South America, is, like yaws and bejel, often acquired in childhood. The primary sore, the 'pintid', appears on the legs. *Treponema carateum,* the cause of pinta, is indistinguishable from *T. pallidum.*

- **Endemic syphilis** occurs when so many people in a community have syphilis that transmission occurs regularly by non-sexual contact. Such a situation existed in Bosnia around the time of World War 2. Primary infection occurs in children and infants, and the disease progresses in the same way as adult infection but, obviously, happens at a younger age. Congenital syphilis is rare in these circumstances because, by the time girls are of childbearing age, the disease has entered the late stage when transmission to the fetus is less likely.

Endemic syphilis was eradicated following an intensive campaign by the World Health Organization, in which everyone at possible risk was given penicillin.

Resources

http://www.bashh.org/guidelines UK National Guidelines.

http://www.iusti.org/regions/Europe/draft_syphilis_leaflet.pdf Patient leaflet on syphilis.

10

Tropical and other infections

→ Key points

- Gay men account for 99% of lymphogranuloma venereum (LGV) in the UK
- Most men (74%) diagnosed with LGV are also infected with HIV
- LGV in heterosexuals can still be imported from tropical countries.

The three 'tropical' diseases, LGV, chancroid and donovanosis, are all associated with warmer climes but, since 2003, LGV has appeared in men who have sex with men (MSM), mostly HIV-positive, in Belgium, Holland, France, and the UK.

What does LGV do?

LGV is caused by the L1–3 serovars of *Chlamydia trachomatis* and affects gay men differently from heterosexuals, reflecting their predominantly rectal route of infection.

The incubation period is usually 1–4 weeks and the first sign is a small transient sore. Because this little ulcer is in the vagina or on the labia in women, it is rarely noticed. Likewise a rectal sore is missed in gay men.

With penile or vaginal infection, there is enlargement of the lymph glands in the groin, a bubo. This painful, usually one-sided, swelling may develop into an abscess discharging pus. Enlarged glands have a concavity between them—the 'sign of the groove'. Women may not develop as marked a bubo as men with penile infection.

Late complications of LGV are more common and more serious in women

In MSM, because the infection starts in the rectum, the lymph drains to glands within the abdominal cavity, so a bubo is rare. The first symptoms are those of a 'proctitis', an inflammation of the rectum: these comprise lower abdominal pain, perianal pain, discharge of blood and mucus, or pus from the rectum. Constipation may follow as a result of the discomfort.

> In the UK, 849 cases of LGV were diagnosed between 2003 and 2008, most of whom had symptoms of proctitis

The late complications of LGV, not yet seen in the gay men's epidemic, result from LGV's blockage of lymph glands and lymphatic channels. Fluid builds up in the tissues causing *chronic lymphatic oedema*. If untreated, this swelling, known as elephantiasis, becomes permanent. In women, the vulva can become grossly enlarged from the clitoris to the anus. An equivalent complication of the male organ is the 'saxophone penis'.

Other complications are more common in women than men and involve the lower bowel, leading to cancer in some cases.

_i_ Patient perspective

Miguel J. was a 37-year-old film editor from Seville who had an 'open' relationship with Claude, his long-term partner. This allowed oral sex with other men but no penetrative sex. Both had tested HIV-negative 2 years previously. Miguel consulted his family doctor after developing pain when he went to the toilet and fresh blood on his underwear.

He was reassured and prescribed some constipation medicine but 5 days later his pain became severe enough to take him to the local hospital. There he was noted to have a high fever and was admitted for 'observation'. The professor of gastroenterology advised a biopsy. Miguel was asked about any family history of bowel conditions and also about recent travel. He had been in Amsterdam 6 weeks previously but this was at least a month before his symptoms had appeared. The biopsy report showed changes compatible with Crohn's disease, an inflammation of the bowel, and appropriate treatment was started.

A chance meeting with a dermatovenereologist colleague alerted the professor to the possibility of LGV and a sample from the bowel tested positive for an 'L' serovar of chlamydia. Unfortunately his HIV test was also positive and it appeared that Miguel had picked up both infections at a gay club in Amsterdam where, although no penile penetration took place, he had allowed insertion of a hand into his rectum ('fisting'), giving an ideal opportunity for infection to be transmitted. Miguel subsequently also tested positive for hepatitis C, bringing to three the total of infections picked up in one night.

How is LGV diagnosed and treated?

In heterosexuals early LGV might be confused with genital herpes, syphilis, chancroid, or donovanosis.

Nowadays proctoscopy, visual examination of the rectum, is an early step for MSM with rectal or anal symptoms. The ordinary tests for *Chlamydia trachomatis* will also pick up LGV, a provisional diagnosis that can be confirmed in a specialist laboratory. A rising or high level of antibodies to LGV in the blood suggests the diagnosis, but sensitivity and specificity of these tests is less than perfect.

> Spread of LGV is facilitated by lack of symptoms—vaginal infection in women and rectal infection in MSM

The treatment of LGV uses the same antibiotics as for non-specific urethritis (NSU), doxycycline, a tetracycline, or macrolides like erythromycin, usually for 3 weeks.

Chancroid

Key facts

* Chancroid used to be the most common cause of genital ulcers in the developing world
* It was isolated from 20 to 60% of patients with genital ulcerations until the early 1990s
* In Africa, ulcers caused by HSV2 are increasing, those due to chancroid are decreasing.

Also called 'soft sore', 'soft chancre', and 'ulcus molle', chancroid is only seen in Western Europe or North America when it has been imported from the main endemic areas of South and East Africa, India, and Caribbean countries. Unlike the chancre of syphilis, the ulcers in chancroid are usually painful and soft, not indurated and hard.

> Chancroid is known to be an important cofactor in the transmission of HIV

The bacterium responsible, *Haemophilus ducreyi*, is hard to find and difficult to culture.

> Chancroid occurs with syphilis or herpes in over 10% of patients in Africa

What does chancroid do?

The sores develop within 7 days of infection. These are acutely painful and, in women, the discomfort is increased by an external dysuria. The infection spreads to the lymph nodes in the groin with bubo formation. If untreated, this swelling eventually breaks down and discharges pus.

> Chancroid is an important cofactor in HIV transmission

How is chancroid diagnosed and treated?

Microscopy only detects 50% of positives found by culture. Other infections, such as herpes, are often also present.

> Men with chancroid outnumber women five to one

Many antibiotics work against chancroid although some antibiotic resistance is being seen.

Donovanosis (granuloma inguinale)

This condition, caused by *Klebsiella granulomatis*, occurs in small pockets around the world, in southern Africa, parts of aboriginal Australia, Papua New Guinea, Brazil, China, and the Caribbean.

The organism is not very infectious and is more common in darker skinned individuals. Only some 50% of sexual partners end up infected, even after prolonged exposure.

What does it do?

The incubation period ranges from a few days to 2 months. A small papule or spot ulcerates and spreads outwards, leaving a raised, velvety reddened area that bleeds easily. It may spread to the perineum, thighs, and buttocks with small nodules under the skin, pseudo-buboes. The area infected enlarges slowly over a period of months. Infection of the cervix looks very much like a carcinoma. At childbirth, caesarean section may be needed to prevent transmission to the baby.

> Because of its low infectivity, it should be possible to eradicate donovanosis

Treatment is with broad spectrum antibiotics, including tetracyclines and azithromycin.

Sexually transmitted diarrhoeal infections

Diarrhoea associated with sex was first reported from the west coast of America in the mid-1970s and given the catchy but inaccurate epithet of the 'gay bowel syndrome', inaccurate because infection depends on sexual behaviour rather than sexual orientation. Anilingus is not restricted to homosexual men any more than is receptive rectal intercourse.

There are three main bacterial causes, one viral and three protozoal:

- Salmonellosis
- Shigellosis
- Campylobacter infection
- Viral hepatitis A (Chapter 11)
- Giardiasis
- Amoebic dysentery
- Cryptosporidiosis.

Each of these diseases is passed on by the faeco–oral route. Normally this describes food poisoning passed on by chefs and other food handlers as a result of poor hygiene. Direct contact of tongue to anus 'cuts out the middle man' and serves as an efficient, direct way of acquiring infection.

Finally, a nematode, *Enterobius vermicularis*, the threadworm, can be passed on during sexual activity. Usually seen in young children with itchy bottoms, it infects an adult just as efficiently.

The infestations

Two infestations are known to be sexually transmitted, 'crabs' and scabies. Neither *has* to be passed on this way indeed, there are outbreaks of scabies in families, nursing homes, nunneries, and hospital wards, but it is rare for crabs to be caught other than during sex.

Phthirus pubis (the crab louse)

Pubic lice, the 'butterflies of love', like their cousins, head and body lice, are insects adapted to a parasitic lifestyle.

Crab lice are almost always sexually transmitted

Very rarely, there is a convincing story of having slept in a soiled bed and catching them that way. *Very rarely*. Crabs cannot live for long away from their human hosts and move very slowly. They do not jump. You can't catch them from a toilet!

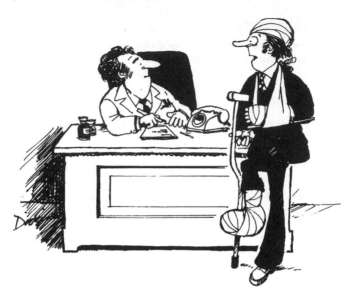

'I did it falling off a lavatory seat.'

The incubation period is between 2 and 4 weeks. The adult female louse takes advantage of close contact, transfers across and begins laying eggs. The 'nits', which are cemented to pubic hairs, hatch, become adults, and start to reproduce. It is not until this cycle has been repeated several times that the sheer number of lice makes their presence known.

What are pubic lice like?

The lice are tiny, not much more than a millimeter in length, flat, and never seem to move when you watch them. The nits are smaller, pinhead-sized, and are laid at the base of a hair. By the time they are ready to hatch, the hair will have grown a little and taken them away from the skin surface.

Pubic lice are generally found only in pubic and perianal hair. Rarely they infect the eyelashes or eyebrows and, in particularly hairy people, infest body hair as well. They are virtually never found in head hair.

What will I notice if I have crabs and how is it diagnosed?

Crab louse infestation causes itching, largely in the pubic area. It may take a day or two of itching before realization dawns that there are little beasts crawling about.

There are usually more females than the relatively promiscuous males. The female lays perhaps three eggs per day. She grabs a hair and deposits some 'cement' to attach the egg. This glue is very powerful and will not be removed by hot water, soaps, or detergents.

> Pubic lice are not carriers of disease

In only about a quarter of cases have the patients actually seen the lice. The itching is not caused by the insects moving but by an allergy to the lice or their faeces. Sometimes faint bluish spots develop at the site of louse bites and scratching may produce a rash.

The crab louse is a natural brown colour and is often difficult to see. They may take on a reddish tinge after feeding on blood.

If lice infest the eyelashes or eyebrows, they cause an inflammation around the eye. Careful examination will reveal the telltale nits attached to the hairs.

What is the treatment?

Virtue's Household Physician of 1924 suggests: 'the main object in the treatment of these filthy diseases is the destruction of the parasite…strict cleanliness of the person is a *sine qua non*…the remedies usually employed are the mercurials, sulphur, carbolic acid, tobacco, etc'. In reality, none of these remedies is effective, and cleanliness, while indeed close to godliness, does not lead to louselessness.

> Two out of five people with crabs will have another sexually transmitted disease

In the old days, DDT gave a reliable cure and benzyl benzoate or gamma-benzene hexachloride were effective. More modern agents include permethrin and malathion, familiar to gardeners as a treatment for greenfly on roses. These products kill both the adult lice and their eggs, but will not remove the nits from the hairs. Shaving, carefully, or a close friend with a fine-toothed comb will do the trick.

The products mentioned above can be harmful if in contact with the eyes—if you think your eyebrows or eyelashes are infested, it is better to go to your GP or a GUM clinic. Treated patients tend to return to clinic after a week or so demanding further treatment because the nits, although dead, remain attached to the hairs.

Scabies (*Sarcoptes scabiei*)

Scabies, the 'Royal itch', is in the list of sexually transmitted infections (STIs) under slightly false pretences. While it *can* be sexually transmitted, it is passed on more frequently non-sexually. The itch is not painful and James the First (hence the 'Royal') claimed that the itch was fit only for kings, so exquisite was his pleasure in scratching.

What causes scabies?

The female of *Sarcoptes scabiei,* var. *hominis,* is 4 mm in length, twice the size of the male. Different mammals have their own varieties of scabietic mite.

Who gets scabies?

Close contact, not necessarily genital, is needed for transmission. Schoolchildren pass it on holding hands, nurses catch it moving patients, and it can infest whole families with ease. Once contact is made with a new host, the mite burrows through the skin and lays eggs. These hatch, emerge on the surface of the skin, copulate, and the females burrow again to repeat the cycle.

Scabies is often passed on 'innocently' between friends and acquaintances

Because the scabies mite prefers loose skin, it favours sites such as finger webs, wrists, breasts, and buttocks and, of course, the skin of the penis and foreskin.

What are the signs and symptoms of scabies?

The main symptom is itching, serious itching, not confined to the genital area but below the head and neck. The cause of the itch is not the mite moving or burrowing, but an allergy to the mite and its excrement. This may take weeks rather than days to develop, by which time cycles of reproduction have taken place and the mite has spread over much of the body.

The itching is so intense that it is almost impossible not to scratch. Scratching leads to secondary bacterial infection and nasty, weeping, swollen sores. If these are on the penis it is not unnatural to assume an awful venereal disease.

How is the diagnosis made?

The history and distribution of the itch, and the sight of the mites' burrows, make a clinical diagnosis easy, particularly if partners or family members are similarly affected. In a GUM clinic, the burrow can be 'de-roofed', an adult mite and/or its eggs hooked out and identified under a microscope.

What is the treatment?

The same products used for crab lice work equally well with scabies. Permethrin, malathion or similar compounds are effective and must be applied to the whole body surface for 12 hours. Because the itch is due to an allergy, killing the mites and their eggs does not get rid of the itch, which may take several days to disappear.

Resources

http://www.iusti.org/regions/Europe/Euro_guideline_LGV_2010.pdf European guidelines on LGV.

http://www.iusti.org/regions/Europe/Draft_Euroguideline_Chancroid 17.05.10.pdf European guidelines on chancroid.

http://www.iusti.org/regions/Europe/Euro_Guideline_Pediculosis_2010.pdf European guidelines on pubic lice.

http://www.iusti.org/regions/Europe/Euro_Guideline_Scabies_2010.pdf European guidelines on scabies.

11

Hepatitis and other viral infections

> ## ⮕ Key points
>
> - Hepatitis A, B, and C are sexually transmitted viruses causing hepatitis
> - Hepatitis A, B, and C can all be caught in a non-sexual way
> - Cytomegalovirus can be sexually transmitted and poses problems in immunocompromised individuals.

Hepatitis A, B, and C

Hepatitis means an '-*itis*', or inflammation, of the liver. There are many causes, some infectious, some chemical, some unexplained. It may seem strange to have a section on hepatitis amongst a host of sexually related conditions, but three viruses, hepatitis A, B, and C, are sexually transmitted under certain circumstances. The third of these, hepatitis C, has only recently joined its two companions as a generally accepted STI.

How do you catch viral hepatitis?

Hepatitis A is transmitted in two different ways:

- Most infections result from eating or drinking something prepared by someone themselves infected with the virus; this is the classical 'food poisoning' form of hepatitis. Outbreaks can centre on a kitchen in a busy restaurant or spread within families
- Transmission can occur directly during sex if mouth or tongue (or hand or finger) touches the anus during sex. These forms of transmission are independent of gender or sexual orientation but are most common in men who have sex with men (MSM).

Hepatitis B does not spread as readily as hep A but is more infectious given the right circumstances—some say that it is 1000 times more infectious than HIV. There are three main ways by which hep B is spread.

- Contaminated blood—all blood and blood products are routinely tested for hep B in the UK and the risk of infection by this means is effectively zero.

However, injecting drug users (IDUs) who share needles or syringes are at particular risk of hep B (and hep C)

◆ Endemic transmission occurs where hep B is common (up to 20% infected), such as Africa, South East Asia, the Mediterranean, Eastern Europe, and Central and South America. Mother-to-baby transmission also occurs

◆ Anal intercourse is an efficient method of transmission, so MSM are especially at risk. Heterosexual transmission occurs in endemic areas.

Hepatitis C transmission is similar to hep B. Hep C is less infectious than hep B.

◆ Blood products—before the 1991 blood test to detect hep C, haemophiliacs and recipients of blood transfusions were at risk; IDUs make up the majority of cases of hep C infection

◆ Sexual transmission is inefficient but, as with hep B, there is a rising prevalence amongst MSM, particularly those with HIV

◆ Mother-to-infant transmission occurs occasionally when the mother is HIV-positive.

What happens with hepatitis?

The average incubation period of hep A is 28 days and most people with hep A recover without further problems. The disease is mild in children and more severe in older folk. Death from hep A is rare and largely occurs in those over 50.

Acute hep B, like A, may produce no symptoms, particularly in children and HIV-positive individuals. For those who do become unwell, the illness may take up to 5 or 6 months to show itself although most cases are diagnosed earlier. The signs and symptoms, for those who develop them, are like those of hep A.

The incubation period of hep C is 1–5 months. There are usually no symptoms when infection occurs and in a majority there will be no indication that infection has taken place.

Between 2005 and 2008, UK reported cases of hep C increased from 6193 to 8563 annually, possibly because of ascertainment bias (see Chapter 2).

Are there any complications of hepatitis?

Hepatitis A is a self-limiting disease that is followed by return to full health and immunity from further attacks. Adults are more likely than children to develop a 'flu-like illness followed by jaundice. A very tiny number develop serious liver failure.

Hepatitis B—in most cases, full health and immunity follow infection. However, in 5–10% of symptomatic patients the virus is not eliminated and a 'carrier' state ensues. Such a state can be infectious (see below), and may lead to liver damage and cirrhosis.

> One in ten of those with cirrhosis due to hep B develop cancer of the liver

Between 50% and 85% of those infected with hep C become chronic carriers of the virus (and therefore potentially infectious to others), with a third going on to permanent liver damage after 20 years or so.

> Only one in 50 long-term partners of those with hep C become infected themselves

How is hepatitis infection diagnosed?

A combination of blood tests can determine whether infection is current, in the past, chronic, or absent, and whether vaccination, in the case of hep A and hep B, is indicated.

Two boring paragraphs on hepatitis B blood tests

Unless you have a personal interest in hepatitis B, you will be forgiven for skipping the following.

Hep B is more complicated than hep A and the blood tests are poorly understood by many doctors and nurses, let alone patients. If somebody has never been infected with hep B and never been vaccinated, there are no antibodies in the blood. Simple. When an infection has occurred in the past (often without symptoms), there will be antibodies to the 'core' of the virus, hepatitis B core antibody, or hep B cAb, for short. If the patient fully recovered, there will also be another test showing antibodies to hepatitis B surface antigen, hep B sAb. All other tests will be negative.

If, however, some viral infection persists, part of the virus itself, the surface antigen, in shorthand, hep B sAg, can be detected. If surface antigen is found, this means active virus is still present in the body and the person in question is infectious, but not greatly so. A further blood test looks for *antibodies* to the 'e' antigen, hep B eAb, also positive in persons of 'low infectivity'. Detection, however, of the 'e' *antigen*, hep B eAg, means very high infectivity, enough to stop a surgeon, for instance, from ever operating again.

The standard antibody test for hep C may take 3 months to become positive. A test that identifies hep C RNA becomes positive 1 month after infection.

Prevention and treatment for hepatitis

Prevention is better than cure and comes in the form of vaccination. Vaccination, like past infection with hepatitis A or B, gives lifelong immunity. There is no vaccine against hep C infection.

Hepatitis A vaccination can be *active*, when a person's immune system is stimulated to make antibodies. One injection is now thought to be enough for permanent immunity.

> *Active* vaccine, if given within 8 days to hep A contacts, prevented infection in 80%. None developed symptoms

Passive immunization against hep A uses human immunoglobulin from someone previously infected.

Hepatitis B—vaccination is recommended for MSM or heterosexual partners of chronic hep B carriers, but not others, in GUM clinics. There is little evidence of significant transmission within low-risk groups.

Those with active hep B or hep C need liver function tests and, if there is evidence of deterioration, may need antiviral agents. In hep C infection, the results of treatment depend on the subtype of virus: genotypes 2 and 3 have a 50% cure rate; other genotypes fare less well.

> Type 1 genotype is more likely to clear spontaneously but leads to more severe chronic infection

Molluscum contagiosum

Molluscum contagiosum (MC) is a viral skin condition that, like scabies, sits somewhat uncomfortably in a list of STIs. It is by no means always sexually transmitted although, like scabies, it *can* be, particularly when the spots are near the genitals. Often MC is passed on innocently by casual, non-sexual, contact. Once present, MC may be spread by scratching or shaving the pubic hair.

Most people suffering from MC are seen by general practitioners or dermatologists.

What are the signs and symptoms of MC?

There is a wide incubation period, from 2 weeks to several months. The spots of MC are pink with a 'pearly' sheen on the top. They vary in size from 2 mm to 1 cm across and number as many as 30 or 40.

In 99.9% of cases the diagnosis is made by the characteristic appearance of the spots, which may itch a little. HIV infection can lead to bad outbreaks of MC on the face.

What is the treatment of MC?

The liquid nitrogen spray used for warts is the standard treatment. Freezing sometimes leaves a small scar or small area of depigmentation.

This is a benign condition that improves without any treatment after some months.

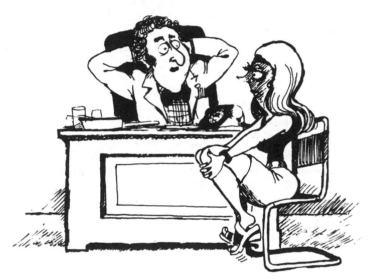

'When I mentioned airborne viruses, I wasn't thinking of a business class flight.'

Cytomegalovirus

Cytomegalovirus (CMV) is a member of the herpes family and causes few problems in those with an intact immune system. Nearly 100% of adults in less developed countries and 50% worldwide are infected.

How is CMV caught?

CMV can be acquired from breast milk or contact with other children. Adults acquire it sexually or by blood transfusion or even organ transplant.

What does CMV do?

In most cases, absolutely nothing. In childhood it may produce no symptoms at all or give an illness similar to glandular fever. In developed countries, primary infection can occur in adults.

CMV's importance is for those with deficient immune systems. Recipients of kidney, liver, or bone marrow transplants have their immunity deliberately reduced to stop rejection. Those with HIV infection are susceptible because of their immunosuppression.

Before highly active antiretroviral therapy (HAART), 25% of people living with AIDS developed CMV in the retina, leading to blindness. Involvement of the nervous system and gastrointestinal tract also occur.

Blood tests help diagnosis and several antiviral drugs are effective, but nowadays good treatment of the HIV infection is the best way to control CMV.

Resources

http://www.bashh.org/guidelines Management of viral hepatitides.

http://www.bashh.org/guidelines Management of molluscum contagiosum.

http://www.hpa.org.uk/web/HPAwebFile/HPAweb_C/1194947317758 HPA information on CMV.

http://www.chelwest.nhs.uk/documents/hiv_factsheets/general/CMV.pdf Patient leaflet on CMV.

12

HIV and AIDS—the whys and wherefores

> ## → Key points
>
> ◆ Worldwide, most human immunodeficiency virus (HIV) is spread by heterosexuals
>
> ◆ The Caribbean has the second highest prevalence after Africa
>
> ◆ HIV is not as infectious as hepatitis B.

Infection with HIV has not spread *evenly* throughout the world, nor *equally* amongst different sections of the human community. The likelihood of catching HIV during a sexual act will depend on geographical and behavioural factors: unprotected vaginal sex with a commercial sex worker carries a greater risk in Lesotho than in Leicester or Lake Placid.

When was HIV first noticed?

An article in the American public health journal (*MMWR*) first brought HIV to the attention of the medical profession in 1981. 'Pneumocystis pneumonia—Los Angeles' centred on a neat piece of detective work by medical epidemiologists, those who measure disease trends. Our sleuths had noticed an increase in requests from Los Angeles for pentamidine, a drug used to treat a lung infection, *Pneumocystis carinii* pneumonia (PCP), which occurs in some patients following kidney transplantation.

Their inquiries revealed that the five treated cases in LA were not transplant patients but men who have sex with men (MSM). Transplant patients develop PCP because their immune system is (deliberately) weakened with drugs to reduce the chances of rejection of their new kidney. However, none of the gay men was taking such medication; their immune system was being weakened in some other way.

> A rare tumour, Kaposi's sarcoma, was also detected in gay men

Within the year more HIV cases had been reported from San Francisco and New York to add to the increasing number in LA. A few sporadic cases had occurred in the UK by the end of 1982, but the large majority were in the USA, most of them in MSM—most of them, but not all.

Who was at risk? The four 'H's

AIDS was seen to be affecting four main groups of people:

- Homosexual men
- Heroin addicts
- Haemophiliacs
- Haitians.

The puzzling thing was not that they all began with 'H', but why Haitians, in the main heterosexual, constituted a risk group. The risk for haemophiliacs and injecting drug users (IDUs) could be explained if there were an infectious agent, probably a virus, in blood and blood products. But Haitians?

> HIV is much less infectious than hepatitis B

The Haitian cases were reported from New York and Miami, both with a large number of Haitian immigrants. The disease was most common in recent immigrants and 30% were women, which didn't fit with the media's label of the new disease as the 'gay compromise syndrome'.

One explanation was that Haiti acted as a staging post in the passage of HIV from Africa to the United States. Zaire, a new nation, had freed itself of Belgian influence and needed French-speaking teachers, civil servants, middle management, and francophone Haiti was chosen.

While most of the Haitians were heterosexual, a few were gay, and Haiti was a popular holiday resort for homosexual New Yorkers. Whatever the connection, once in the States, spread was rapid, with one well documented progression of HIV from a New York gay man to several contacts on the West Coast.

Where did HIV come from?

HIV infection originated in the continent of Africa.

HIV infection is neither a result of some grim CIA plan to take over the world, nor was it spread through Africa by polio immunizations in the 1980s. Conspiracy theorists have produced such explanations for the global pandemic but the truth is simpler, if less attractive to those with a political rather than a scientific agenda.

> Human immunodeficiency virus evolved from simian immunodeficiency virus, SIV

The first infection of a man or woman with HIV must have occurred decades before cases were recognized in the USA in 1981. HIV is very similar to SIV, which infects chimpanzees in Africa. It is possible to work out, using mathematical back-tracking, how long it would have taken for SIV to change to HIV. This happened in the earlier part of the twentieth century, some 60 years before AIDS first emerged in America.

> HIV2 is similar to SIV found in the *sooty mangabey* in West Africa

HIV changes rapidly, explaining why it has proved so difficult to make an effective vaccine and how it develops resistance to antiviral drugs so rapidly.

Why did it spread so fast?

The chances of transmitting HIV depend, amongst other things, on:

- **Behaviour**—injecting HIV directly into the bloodstream as happens with factor VIII or an IDU's syringe, is the most efficient. Rectal intercourse is riskier than vaginal intercourse, which is riskier than oral sex
- **Viral load**—transmission occurs more readily when there are more viruses, as during the 'seroconversion' period just after infection.

If HIV is introduced to a group of people who are frequently sharing risk, most will be seroconverting with a high viral load, making transmission that much more efficient.

Two examples:

- In the late 1970s and early 1980s, there existed in California a notorious 'bath-house' scene for gay men. Alcohol and recreational drugs abounded, and casual couplings were the order of the day and night. I was told by some of my British patients who had been to San Francisco around that time that three partners per night was not unusual. *Every night.* Hundreds of sexual contacts a year. Introduce HIV into that scenario and it will spread rapidly
- The increase amongst needle sharing in IDUs in Edinburgh in the early 1980s saw the prevalence of HIV infection rise from 1.5% in 1983 to 55% in 1985.

So, those who are seroconverting are more likely to pass on HIV because of more virus. If HIV infection is not controlled by antiretroviral drugs, the viral load and infectiousness begin to rise again. Viral load also begins to go up when other infections like tuberculosis or meningitis occur. Other STIs provoke excretion of more virus and make the person more infectious.

Who catches HIV infection?

The simple answer, and that loved by the propagandists of the 1980s, is that *anyone* can. It is certainly true that anybody *can*, but not everybody *does*. Further, different people seem at different risk in different parts of the world. I deal with the various risk groups and risk activities in the order in which they emerged and became apparent.

- The first epidemic to be described in detail was that in **MSM** in the USA. They remain the largest group to suffer from HIV/AIDS on that continent. Likewise, the first cases in the UK and in Europe were found in gay men

- **Injecting drug users**, IDUs, who share equipment, come a close second in numbers in the USA to MSM. The expected increase in IDUs with HIV in western Europe has not happened, but this risk group predominates in eastern Europe and parts of the Far East

- The risk of HIV infection in **haemophiliacs** was high in the days before the antibody test for HIV. New infections, like those from blood transfusions, are virtually unheard of today

- Bisexual men initially seen as a potential 'bridge' from high-risk groups into the general population, have not been numerically important apart from in Central and South American countries where the 'macho' culture frowns on open homosexuality. MSM may marry to mask their preferred sexual orientation

- **Heterosexuals**—worldwide, heterosexual cases outnumber all the other categories put together. Sub-Saharan Africa has the largest number of sufferers of HIV/AIDS, almost exclusively heterosexual.

So, risk activities are associated with risk groups, but closer analysis shows an uneven spread of infection even within the different groupings. Do all heroin addicts have an equal risk of infection? Are all gay men as likely to catch HIV? Is the probability of infection the same for all heterosexuals in Africa or, for that matter, in Seattle, in Trinidad, or in the UK? The answer to all these questions is 'No'.

Throughout the world there are racial and ethnic differences in rates of infection owing to local circumstances, behavioural differences, and simple factors such as the provision and uptake of healthcare.

In the UK it took some time for this politically incorrect, differential risk to be accepted, with the result that neither heterosexual positives (predominantly black) nor gay men (predominantly white) received the targeted healthcare or health advice that should have been theirs, until well into the 1990s.

> Worldwide, 'needlestick' infection, passed on by pricking or cutting with a contaminated needle or scalpel, is rare.

The epidemic in the USA

Although the first report of PCP in five gay men was published in the *MMWR* in 1981, the epidemic must have been around at least during the 1970s in the USA since it took around 10 years to develop AIDS after initial HIV infection.

In America the number of cases associated with Africa made up a lower proportion than in Europe, but the IDU numbers were higher. A blood test became available in 1984 which identified antibodies to HIV in blood, following the identification of the virus responsible for AIDS.

The 'possible' virus had been named HTLV-III by Robert Gallo, an American expert in retroviruses. He published details of this virus in 1983, to worldwide scientific acclaim, at much the same time as did a French virologist, Luc Montagnier, whose laboratory was at the *Institut Pasteur* in Paris. A public scandal ensued when it transpired that the virus 'discovered' by Gallo was identical to one that Montagnier had sent him previously, as a courtesy. The virus was renamed HIV in 1986.

❌ Myths

'It's everybody's equal risk' **Untrue**

'Oral sex carries a high risk of HIV' **Untrue**

'Having sex with a virgin is a cure for HIV' (from Africa) **Untrue**

The San Francisco General Hospital modelled its care on keeping infected individuals out of hospital. There was also a keen desire to involve patients in their own care and be part of any decision-making process.

In the UK at the time, many physicians were unhappy with the suggestion that a patient should be told about, let alone asked for permission for, an HIV test. 'Damn it, we don't discuss haemoglobin tests or cancer investigations...' was a typical reaction. Probably the only good thing to have come out of the HIV epidemic was this change, prompted by the positive gay community, in the degree of patient involvement, not just those with HIV, in decisions about their own health.

The epidemic in America has progressed from a predominantly male homosexual one to high numbers of drug-related cases and a significant proportion of heterosexually acquired infections. As in the UK, it is ethnic minorities, in this case African-American and Hispanic, who are disproportionately involved, as are an increasing number of women.

- African-American men are 6.5 times more likely to develop HIV than Caucasian men in the USA
- African-American women are 19 times more likely to develop HIV than Caucasian white women in the USA

In New York City women are twice as likely to be infected by a husband or steady boyfriend as by a casual sex partner. However, the majority of persons alive and HIV-infected in the USA remain MSM.

It is worth repeating that race and ethnicity are not in themselves risk factors for HIV. Poverty and socioeconomic deprivation are strongly related to risk. Up-to-date figures and breakdowns of risk groups can be found at the UNAIDS website.

The epidemic in the UK

The Communicable Disease Surveillance Centre (CDSC) is the UK equivalent of the Centers for Disease Control in the USA and, like the CDC, has been responsible for collecting HIV/AIDS figures since the start of the epidemic.

As in America, the British epidemic started with MSM. British gay men had been envious of the uncluttered, free approach to sex on the West Coast and, by mid-1983, seven of the first 12 MSM AIDS cases had had sex with men in the USA. The only haemophiliac case had used factor VIII from America

It was accepted, after a struggle, that supplying clean needles and syringes to IDUs was the obvious way to reduce person-to-person transmission, and needle exchange facilities became increasingly available. *Moralists* complained that, by doing so, society was not only condoning misuse of drugs but encouraging it. *Realists* just got on with reducing infection rates.

By the end of 1986 the increasing number of infected heterosexuals was to become the focus of much attention and provide propaganda for safer sex in the general population.

Was the British public misled about the heterosexual risk?

In late 1986 an interesting change occurred in the way heterosexual cases were reported.

Until then, most of the heterosexuals in the CDSC's monthly HIV reports were identified by a footnote '…associated with sub-Saharan Africa'. This footnote was missing from tables published in November 1986, and heterosexual AIDS cases were simply subdivided into 'presumed infected abroad' and 'presumed infected UK'. The December HIV tables lost even that distinction and simply referred to 'heterosexuals'.

This change in reporting categories happened 1 month before a nationwide leaflet drop, in January 1987, to every household in the UK, part of the campaign: '**AIDS—Don't Die of Ignorance**'.

The increasing number of heterosexual cases was emphasized and most people, encouraged by the media, assumed that heterosexual cases *reported* in the UK were the same as heterosexual cases *transmitted* in the UK. Those infected in sub-Saharan Africa were assumed to be UK nationals who had travelled there, rather than citizens of African countries.

This loss of the 'African connection' in the reported figures lasted until the early 1990s, with two important consequences. It convincingly supported the myth of an ever-increasing epidemic of heterosexual HIV *transmission* in the UK, and it denied health targeting to a particularly vulnerable section of the community in Great Britain. Although the figures have been quite transparent since the mid-1990s, each year the media still talk of the massive HIV epidemic as if *transmission* is occurring predominantly in the UK.

What then is the truth?

The figures are freely available from the website of the Health Protection Agency.

The majority of heterosexuals in the UK with HIV/AIDS acquired their infection in sub-Saharan Africa and, of the new cases reported each year, only a small proportion were actually caught in the UK from someone themselves infected in the UK. An unknown percentage of the total will be infections passed in the UK between persons from a high-risk area.

New heterosexual HIV transmissions 2008

		UK transmissions
Reported new cases of HIV in the UK	**3862**	3862
850 No details	3862 minus 850	= 3012
1774 Acquired in Africa	3012 minus 1774	= 1238
367 Acquired elsewhere outside UK	1238 minus 367	= 871
341 Partners MSM/IDU/other risk/not known	871 minus 341	= 530
313 Partners infected in Africa (59%)	530 minus 313	= **217**

The above table, adapted from the HPA's published figures, shows how the numbers are open to misinterpretation. Excluding transmissions by injecting drug abusers (166) and mother-to-baby (99), there were 3862 new cases of HIV in heterosexuals reported in the UK for 2008. But, subtracting the 850 without details and all others with any risk factors, we are left with a final total of only 217 definitely no-risk individuals.

So should we be complacent about heterosexual transmission of HIV in the UK? Absolutely not. We have been spared the degree of infection seen elsewhere, perhaps because of a (comparatively) low level of other STDs found in the UK helped by the provision of a network of clinics throughout the country, free at the point of access.

What of the other risk categories? Since 1994 there has been an average of 30 new blood factor cases annually and new IDU infections were 166 in 2008, of which 59 were from the UK. Mother-to-infant cases, a reflection on the heterosexual epidemic, peaked at 144 cases in 2003 and were 99 for 2008.

Since the year 2000 there has been a steady increase (75%) in HIV infection amongst gay men. This has attracted little notice since the figures have been overshadowed by the increase in heterosexual cases. There is a suggestion that some gay men are ignoring the lessons of the past and ditching safer sex practices because of the greatly improved outlook for those with HIV since the advent of highly active antiretroviral therapy (HAART). (see figure 12.1)

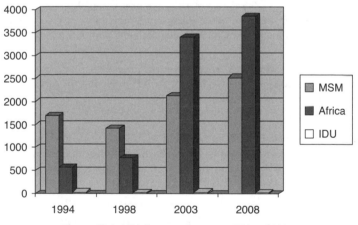

Figure 12.1 HIV diagnoses between 1994 and 2008.

A recent patient of mine, just down from university, was shocked by the sight, in a gay club, of couples openly 'bare-backing'. When we know how well condoms prevent transmission of HIV and other STIs, he found it extraordinary that such risks were being taken, and so openly.

The epidemic in Africa

There are several epidemics of HIV infection in Africa. Some have almost burnt themselves out while others are yet to reach their peak.

According to UNAIDS, sub-Saharan Africa still had the highest worldwide HIV/AIDS burden in 2008, with 67% of all the new HIV infections and 72% of HIV-related deaths

The 'epicentre' of HIV1 infection was thought to be in the region of the Central African Republic and Zaire. There was more rapid spread eastwards and south-wards to Uganda, Kenya, Tanzania, and Zambia. Today, Botswana, Lesotho, and Swaziland all have the highest HIV prevalence, around 25%, with Zimbabwe, South Africa, Zambia, and Malawi between 10 and 20%.

In Lesotho in 2008, 50% of new HIV infections occurred in steady sexual relationships

The UK cases of HIV originating in Africa (with the exception of the Central African Republic and Zaire) reflect Britain's past colonial history. There is a similar relationship between other European countries in respect of the geo-graphical origin of many cases, for instance, Belgium with Zaire, or France with the Ivory Coast.

Estimates in 2004 suggested that 2.5% of HIV infections in Africa were a result of contaminated needles

Why the disease has grabbed such a hold in Africa has puzzled investigators. In the late 1980s, transmission of HIV was shown to increase when there was a concurrent STD. A study in Mwanza demonstrated a reduction in HIV transmission when a good STI service was instituted.

In Uganda and Zimbabwe, HIV seroconversion was strongly associated with *Trichomonas vaginalis* infection

There are, on average in Africa, 13 HIV-infected women for each 10 men; for those younger than 25 years, the ratio is 36 to 10; in Ghana the figure is more than 9 to 1.

In one study from Zimbabwe and South Africa, two-thirds of women reported having had only one lifetime partner, and four out of five had waited until 17 before having sex (just about the world average), and four out of five said they had used a condom. Yet 40% were HIV-positive.

> In Kenya in 2007, HIV infection was three times more common (13.2%) in uncircumcised than in circumcised men (3.9%)

The epidemic in Europe—east and west

The early epidemic was similar to that in the US and the UK, with a predominance of cases among MSM. Imported cases from Africa made up the majority of heterosexual cases, although injecting drug use was more a feature in the more southern countries, France, Germany, Spain, Italy, and Greece.

In London in the 1980s, more IDUs diagnosed with HIV infection had been born in Italy than in Britain. Those countries that, like the UK, made needle exchange facilities available, diminished transmission significantly.

The figures for central Europe, other than Poland, have remained fairly steady since the late 1990s, but the same is not true of eastern Europe. There are alarming rates of increase in HIV in the Ukraine and the Russian Federation which have paralleled the increase in cases of infectious syphilis, although the HIV epidemic is driven by IDUs. One estimate suggests that between 1 and 2% of the entire Russian population inject drugs.

The epidemic in Asia

The potential for spread and devastation in Asia, home to 60% of the world's population, is hugely greater than sub-Saharan Africa, home to only 10%.

HIV has been well and long established in Thailand, Myanmar, and Cambodia, as well as in parts of India. Vietnam, Indonesia, Nepal, and some provinces in China are just beginning their expansion while others, Sri Lanka, Pakistan, and Bangladesh, for instance, maintain low levels of prevalence, so far.

There is widespread ignorance in China about preventive measures—in one survey from 2003 it was found that 40% of men and women were unable to name a single way in which they could protect themselves from HIV infection.

India now contributes 50% of all Asian HIV infection, with half or more sex workers found to be positive in some states. The contribution of MSM is smaller than in the west, but a high proportion also report sex with women.

In Nepal, Bangladesh, and Vietnam the epidemic is drug-driven, with widespread use of unsterile injecting equipment.

> Women in Vietnam made up 19% of positives in 2000, but 35% of positives in 2008

In Cambodia and Thailand the HIV incidence rate is coming down as condom usage is going up. Education, education, education are needed elsewhere: in Pakistan, with no significant epidemic as yet, one in three lorry drivers had never heard of condoms and in East Timor four of ten sex workers did not recognize a condom when shown one. Education can work:

> Between 2003 and 2006, HIV prevalence among female sex workers in India fell from 10.3% to 4.9%

The epidemic in the Middle East and North Africa

There were about 35 000 new HIV infections in the Middle East and North Africa in 2008. The worst affected area is southern Sudan, where the prevalence of HIV is about 1%, representing more than four in five of all infections in this whole region. One study from Rumbek, in the south, revealed that only one in five people had ever heard of a condom and less than 2% used a condom with a casual sexual partner.

According to UNAIDS in 2009:

◆ Many MSM in the Middle East and North Africa are bisexual

◆ Only 15% of MSM in Jordan use a condom in penetrative anal sex

◆ A high proportion of MSM are also IDUs.

In Libya, Tunisia, and Egypt, there are few infections, mostly in IDUs. Needle exchange programmes are urgently needed. In Morocco, heterosexual intercourse appears to be the main route of transmission. Elsewhere, in Algeria, Bahrain, Oman, and Kuwait, IDU is the major risk factor, as it is in Iran where dramatic increases in HIV numbers have occurred. In part this may be because of ascertainment bias (increased testing for HIV).

Country (2008)	HIV in drug injectors (%)
Oman	11.8
Morocco	6.5
Israel	2.6
Egypt	2.6
Turkey	2.6

Mixing of cultures and countries is inevitable in the oil-rich states and Saudi Arabia provides an example. Most of the HIV-positive cases in Sri Lanka are in young women who have worked in service in the Middle East. They have all tested HIV-negative before leaving their home country, but many return infected as a result of relationships with other immigrant labour, often construction workers from African countries. They contract HIV infection and in some cases pass this on to their employers who sexually abuse them.

The epidemic in Oceania

The majority of transmissions in Australia and New Zealand are between MSM. The small number of cases in heterosexuals has, rather like the UK, occurred in those who come from, or who have had sex in, countries with a high prevalence of heterosexual infection. Aboriginal peoples in Australia have higher than average rates of HIV and other STIs.

Papua New Guinea contributes 95% of the new HIV island diagnoses (New Caledonia 1.2%; French Polynesia 1.1%; Fiji 1.1%; Guam 0.8%; others 0.8%). Antenatal prevalence was around 2% in 2003 and, since then, more new infections have been reported in women than men. Spread is largely fuelled by commercial sex workers. Other Pacific islands have not yet experienced HIV epidemics, but the high rates of other STIs suggest a fertile field.

The epidemic in the Caribbean

The Caribbean is an HIV/AIDS disaster erupting before our eyes. Over the whole region 1.0% of adults are HIV-positive, and AIDS is the most common cause of death amongst those aged between 15 and 44. Many of the islands with the highest rates of HIV infection have popular and developed tourism industries, including Jamaica, the Dominican Republic, Trinidad and Tobago, the Bahamas, Barbados, and Bermuda. The epidemic is largely fuelled by heterosexual transmission, with potential for spread beyond the region's geographical boundaries.

> The Caribbean has the second highest *rate* of HIV infection after Africa

Bermuda and Puerto Rico are the only countries with a significant infection rate amongst IDUs (up to 50% in each).

Haiti featured early in the unfolding story of global HIV spread (see above), and its position with the worst HIV prevalence has been supplanted by the Bahamas, at 3%.

As happened in sub-Saharan Africa, the rate of infection in women has overtaken that in men, with teenage girls more than twice as likely to be infected as boys in parts of the region. Jamaica is one such country and has the second highest number of cases and deaths from AIDS, after Haiti.

In the Caribbean in 2004, only 10% of those needing antiretroviral drugs were in receipt of them, a figure that had reached 51% by 2008

Cuba has avoided the rapid increase in cases seen elsewhere by a combination of strict quarantine rules (since abandoned) and ready availability of healthcare and antiretroviral drugs. The new cases that have been seen have been mostly in homosexual men.

The HIV/AIDS epidemic in the Caribbean will impinge increasingly on those countries which have historical, colonial connections, for instance Surinam with Holland, Montserrat with France, and Jamaica with the UK.

Latin America

Latin America, with 170 000 new HIV cases in 2008, comes third after sub-Saharan Africa (1.9 million) and South East Asia (280 000) in total numbers.

Bisexuality is more common in this region, with a resulting bridge to the heterosexual population. Many MSM do not think of themselves as homosexual.

- ◆ 17% of MSM in El Salvador, which has the highest HIV prevalence in Central America, regard themselves as heterosexual
- ◆ 22% of MSM in Central America also have sex with women

The sex ratio in Latin America remains tilted strongly towards men, a result of the high number of MSM infections.

Resources

http://www.unaids.org For world figures.

http://www.hpa.org.uk For UK figures.

Erwin JT, Smith DK, Peters BS (eds) (2003) Ethnicity and HIV: Prevention and Cure in Europe and the USA. London, Atlanta: International Press.

13

HIV and AIDS—the clinical picture

➡ Key points

- Early diagnosis of HIV infection makes a full and long life possible
- Treatment of an HIV-positive pregnant woman can eliminate transmission to the baby
- Unprotected sex between two HIV-positive people carries risks.

We have the benefit today of nearly 30 years of clinical experience with HIV infection and can treat or forestall most of the previously life-threatening infections and tumours that affected early sufferers.

In 1997 the concept of 'highly active antiretroviral therapy' (HAART) was born.

HAART combines three different drugs from two different classes and makes it difficult for a highly suppressed virus to mutate enough to develop resistance. Most drug combinations now are once or twice daily.

The advent of HAART made HIV a manageable condition from which people should not die.

For most of the estimated 33 million people living with HIV, universal access remains a dream. By the end of 2008, only 4 million were on treatment out of 9 million needing it.

How is HIV caught?

HIV transmission occurs in a number of *preventable* ways.

Horizontally:

- Sexual contact (the major route of HIV acquisition)
- Blood transfusion or contaminated needles.

Vertically (mother-to-child) during:

- Pregnancy, labour, and delivery
- Breastfeeding.

Screening blood products, needle exchange programmes, post-exposure prophylaxis (PEP), and HAART use in pregnant women have reduced HIV transmission.

What do I do if I have been exposed to HIV?

PEP is the provision of HAART to prevent HIV and must be started within 72 hours of possible exposure. It is continued for 1 month and is available in accident and emergency departments or the genitourinary medicine (GUM) clinic.

Time is of the essence!

> Use of PEP does not lead to an increase in subsequent risk behaviour.

Does PEP work?

Studies using macaque monkeys and the prevention of mother-to-child transmission of HIV in pregnancy (a PEP effect on the baby) suggest it is effective. An 81% reduction in seroconversion in healthcare workers with needlestick exposure, compared to those not treated, is also good evidence. PEP, although an unproven clinical intervention, is recommended on a case-by-case basis.

> The cost of PEP is minimal compared to the £0.5–1.0 million cost of an HIV transmission.

Who should take PEP?

PEP should be taken in those who have had:

- Unprotected vaginal or anal sex with a known HIV-positive person
- Unprotected sex with high-risk individuals
- Condom accidents in any of the above situations
- Needlestick injury from an HIV patient, or sexual assault.

The grimness of the treatment may outweigh the risk of acquiring HIV. PEP may not be required if the contact is receiving HAART and has a fully suppressed viral load.

Should treatment be given early in confirmed primary HIV infection?

British guidelines suggest early treatment if the individual is immunocompromised or has severe symptoms of seroconversion. However, the optimal duration of treatment is unknown. Giving HAART at seroconversion could reduce HIV transmission during this hyperinfectious period.

When considering treatment, we have to take into account the potential side effects of the drugs and the risk of the development of resistant virus if adherence to the medication is poor.

How likely am I to catch HIV from someone who is positive?

Overall, the risk of HIV transmission following a single sex act is low compared with other sexually transmitted infections (STIs) (see figure 13.1). The risk from a single contact depends upon the infectiousness of the HIV-positive individual (HIV viral load, stage of HIV infection, and STIs) and the susceptibility to HIV of their sexual partner, which includes nature and frequency of sexual exposure, and presence of concurrent STIs.

HIV viral load is the single most important determinant in predicting transmission. Early HIV infection is 10 times more infectious than later stages of infection— a problem since most people at this stage are unaware of their infection.

> STIs, including genital ulcer disease, gonorrhoea, and *Trichomonas* have been associated with HIV transmission

Estimates of transmission risks per act

Receptive anal intercourse*	1 in 30–1 in 200
Insertive anal intercourse*	1 in 500–1 in 1000
Receptive vaginal intercourse*	1 in 500–1 in 1000
Insertive vaginal intercourse*	1 in 1000–1 in 5000
Mucous membrane splash*	1 in 1000
Insertive oral sex: likely to be*	1 in 5000 or lower
Receptive oral sex*	1 in 2000 or lower
Needle sharing	1 in 150
Needlestick injury in health workers	1 in 300

* Circumcision and condom use reduces transmission rates for all types of sexual activity.

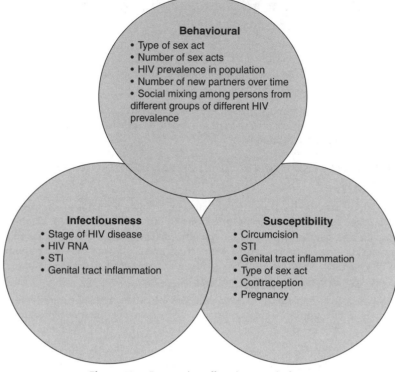

Figure 13.1 Factors that affect the spread of HIV.

Should I have an HIV test?

In the early 1980s there were fears in the gay community of marginalization and victimization at work. Insurance companies upped the premiums for young single men and just taking a test, whatever the result, made you part of a high-risk group and therefore uninsurable.

Since 1989 the Association of British Insurers has advised no increased insurance premiums for those taking HIV tests

Nowadays, with HAART, there is every reason to test.

Put simply, there are two sorts of HIV-positive persons in the west today: those who haven't tested and will die of AIDS, and those who have tested and will die of old age.

What is the 'window period'?

This is the time between catching HIV and the blood test becoming positive. This used to be up to 3 months and many people were advised to wait the full 3 months before testing. Some of today's (fourth generation) HIV tests look for bits of the virus itself and in almost all cases will give an accurate answer after 4 weeks. Check which test you are having so that you can understand the window period.

> After an HIV diagnosis, a second, confirmatory HIV antibody test is mandatory

Early diagnosis is a good thing:

- It allows a person to come to terms with their diagnosis well before needing HAART (which will mean that they will take the treatment better)
- HAART can be started well before the immune system is damaged
- It encourages testing of contacts
- It motivates an individual not to pass on the virus.

ⓘ Patient perspective

John P. was a 55-year-old office worker who turned up at his local A&E complaining of tiredness, weight loss, and shortness of breath. His wife and two grown-up children had come with him. He had a high temperature, a dry cough, was tired, and had lost weight. On admission he was found to have low levels of oxygen in his blood. Pneumonia was diagnosed and antibiotics were started. These had little effect and his condition deteriorated. When the chest X-ray was reviewed, one of his doctors wondered if there was any chance of underlying immune suppression such as HIV.

The doctors raised this possibility with John, who said that he and his wife had not had sex for many years but that he occasionally had sex with men. His HIV test was positive. With appropriate treatment he made a quick recovery from his pneumocystis pneumonia (PCP) and was discharged 10 days later with outpatient follow up. He started antiretroviral therapy 3 weeks later. He told his wife of his diagnosis and she underwent testing and was found to be negative.

How is HIV infection monitored?

Before we start, some of the terms need explaining.

The **CD4 count** (number of CD4 T-helper lymphocytes) reflects how well your immune system is working. In general, more is better. In a healthy person

119

without HIV infection, the CD4 count is 500–1400 mm^3. A CD4 count of less than 200 mm^3 represents severe immunosuppression which may lead to 'opportunistic' i nfections.

The **viral load** measures the number of virus particles in the blood (or other fluid). It is expressed in 'copies per millilitre', often expressed as a 'viral load of 50'. The higher the viral load, the more infectious the individual.

The most important test is the CD4 count because it determines when HAART needs to be started. Current guidelines suggest that this should be at around 350 mm^3, or when the person has symptoms or is coinfected with hepatitis B or C.

British HIV Association treatment guidelines 2008

CD4 <200	Treat
CD4 201–350	Treat soon
CD4 351–500	Treat in certain cases
CD4 >500	Consider 'when to start trial'

Once on HAART, the viral load should be *undetectable* (below 50). A *detectable* viral load suggests failure of treatment or development of drug resistance. If so, the regime may need to be changed.

The aim of HIV management is to keep the patient well. Every 3–6 months patients' emotional and physical welfare are assessed and monitored.

How does HIV infection progress?

Treatment has improved so much over the past 10 years that HIV has become more like a chronic medical problem, such as diabetes, with the important proviso, of course, that HIV is infectious.

The rate of progression of HIV varies between individuals, and is dependent on the severity of the primary infection, lifestyle factors, and the type of HIV acquired. Without treatment, the average time from infection to profound immunosuppression is 10 years. HIV divides into:

- *Early infection*, when the disease lies latent and an infected person appears quite healthy
- *Symptomatic infection*, when illnesses, not AIDS, appear, but there is a measurable immunodeficiency; and, finally
- *Late infection*, when immunosuppression and the risk of a serious infection or tumour (both AIDS-defining illnesses) are greatest.

Early infection

What are the symptoms of seroconversion?

Seroconversion occurs between 5 days and 5 weeks after exposure. Most people are unaware that they have been infected with HIV because symptoms (present in 90%) are non-specific, including fever, sore throat, enlarged lymph nodes, skin rashes, tiredness, and achy joints and muscles.

> The symptoms of HIV seroconversion are much like 'flu

Patients rarely seek medical help and the symptoms settle without any treatment. They rarely warrant admission to hospital.

> Many cases of HIV seroconversion are missed since different viral illnesses, including glandular fever, present in a similar way.

Asymptomatic HIV infection

Following seroconversion, there may be no symptoms or outward signs of HIV for many months or years. Although the CD4 may be above 350 mm^3 and the patient symptom-free, the immune system can become compromised during this time, hence the importance of the 3–6-monthly review. This allows treatment to be offered as soon as it is needed.

As well as regular monitoring, general measures to optimize health and wellbeing are important; these include stopping smoking.

Should I use herbal remedies?

Long-term use of certain herbal remedies, including echinacea, astragalus, and ginseng, should be avoided in people living with HIV. While these substances are claimed to be 'immune enhancers', they might actually enhance virus replication in HIV-positive people.

Do other viruses make HIV worse?

Coinfection with hepatitis B or C and HIV makes progression of each virus faster. Vaccination for hepatitis B and A should be undertaken in all HIV-infected people (if there is no evidence of previous infection).

Risk reduction includes avoiding hepatitis C, other strains of HIV virus, and STIs.

Good HIV management prevents further illness and prevents transmission to other people.

> ## ⓘ Patient perspective
>
> Susan H. presented to the antenatal clinic when 14 weeks pregnant. She had been diagnosed HIV-positive 5 years previously and had not injected drugs for 10 years. Her CD4 count was good, over 500.
>
> Care was coordinated between the midwife, her obstetrician, and her HIV doctor. Her immune system was functioning well but, at week 24 antiretroviral therapy (ART) was started to reduce the risk of transmission to her baby. A date was planned for her caesarean section and it was explained she shouldn't breastfeed. The baby would be given ART for the first 6 weeks of its life.
>
> The pregnancy went well, as did a caesarean section at 38 weeks. Tests on the baby at day 1, and at 6 and 12 weeks, were all negative and the baby is definitely not infected. She did not breastfeed and stopped her drugs after the birth.

Symptomatic HIV infection

The first problems are often minor, with a wide variety of complaints, none pointing to HIV as the underlying diagnosis. The CD4 count might be 200–350 mm^3. Common conditions include oral candida (thrush), persistent skin complaints including eczema, seborrhoeic dermatitis, warts and herpes, recurrent chest infections and mouth ulcers, night sweats, weight loss, gum disease, and fatigue.

> Once symptoms appear, the most important measure is to commence antiretroviral treatment as soon as possible

Recurrent herpes can be treated with daily aciclovir, dry skin with antifungal creams, and oral thrush with antifungal tablets or suspension. We recommend regular dentist/hygienist appointments for gum and tooth complaints.

Late HIV infection

If a patient's CD4 count is less than 200 mm^3, there is marked immunosuppression and a high risk of opportunistic infection (OI) or tumour, which mean that 'AIDS' is present. In the pre-HAART days, an AIDS diagnosis indicated a very poor prognosis with, at best, severe ill-health.

The commonest opportunistic infection is PCP (*Pneumocystis carinii* pneumonia). This fungal infection affects the lungs and presents with a dry cough, fevers, weight loss, and shortness of breath on exertion. Symptoms vary in severity but come on insidiously and gradually.

The 'C' in PCP has recently been renamed 'jiroveci', but 'PJP' has yet to catch on and most use the old name

A number of opportunistic tumours occur, including lymphoma and Kaposi's sarcoma (KS). KS is associated with human herpes virus 8 (HHV8) and can affect any part of the body, but commonly presents with distinctive dusky red papules on the skin. Treatment for the underlying HIV may be enough, but local radiotherapy or chemotherapy is sometimes needed.

Management of late HIV infection

Any patient presenting late needs urgent investigation and management, which often means hospital admission. The underlying condition, PCP for instance, needs confirming with tests and then fully treating *before* any anti-HIV treatment is commenced. Immediate treatment with HAART in these circumstances can do more harm than good. The OI can, paradoxically, actually be worsened by restoring the immune system. HAART is started about 3 weeks after the OI has been treated.

HAART started at a low CD4 count is less effective than starting when the CD4 count is higher. Early diagnosis and treatment is best!

The multidisciplinary approach

It is important to remember to see the person as a whole and address all aspects of their physical and emotional wellbeing, including their sex life. This means helping people to adjust to their diagnosis.

The multidisciplinary model of care includes many individuals: doctors, specialist HIV pharmacists, adherence nurses, research nurses, dieticians, midwives, and counsellors. Strong links with the GUM clinic, support groups, and local advice centres are important.

HAART has improved the prognosis of those with HIV, resulting in a large increase in numbers attending clinics

For individuals with complex problems, on-site availability of other specialties improves the quality of care. Eye, chest, and skin specialists, neurologists, ENT surgeons, and dentists all have their part to play. However, for individuals stable on HAART with no problems (a significant proportion of patients nowadays), follow up in the community is recommended with referral back to tertiary services when needed.

What are the treatments for HIV?

The oldest class of drugs is the **NRTIs**, or nucleoside reverse transcriptase inhibitors, and includes zidovudine, didanosine, lamivudine, abacavir, and emtricitabine (FTC). Tenofovir is a nucleo*tide* reverse transcriptase inhibitor which works in a similar way to NRTIs.

The first drug used for the treatment of HIV was zidovudine (AZT) in the mid-1980s. Originally developed as an anti-cancer therapy, AZT had been shelved because of its bad side effects. It was, however, better than placebo in symptomatic individuals. Although it was not possible to measure at the time, this use of a solitary antiretroviral was a recipe for HIV resistance. For all its drawbacks, AZT provided the first glimmer of hope and certainly prolonged life, albeit for a short time.

> Tenofovir, as a vaginal gel inserted before sex, reduced transmission of HIV by 54%, when used consistently over 2½ years. It also reduced herpes transmission.

The search was on for other NRTIs to replace 'monotherapy' with 'dual therapy' (zidovudine with didanosine, lamivudine, or zalcitabine). These combinations reduced mortality by 36% over a 3-year period.

Non-nucleoside reverse transcriptase inhibitors (**NNRTIs**) are drugs that only work on HIV1, not HIV2. There are NNRTIs, namely efavirenz, nevirapine, and, more recently, etravirine, to which resistance develops less readily.

With the arrival of this second class of drugs, the era of *triple* therapy had begun, making tight control of HIV infection possible.

However, HIV is capable of changing and developing resistance very rapidly. Nevirapine, for instance, becomes rapidly useless on its own or as one of a pair. This is one of the most important messages of HIV therapy.

Every effort must be made to prevent development of resistance.

This means that adequate amounts of drug must be given and treatment must be taken without fail.

Easy enough, you might think, but, in the early days of triple therapy there was a real burden simply in managing to take all the drugs (more than 30 a day in some cases) on certain regimens. In others, the side effects were really difficult to cope with.

In 1996, another class of drugs was introduced, the **protease inhibitors** (PIs), which bind to one of the virus's enzymes and stop further replication. These had a massive effect on survival. Initially difficult to take, they have improved partly because they are coadministered with ritonavir which improves their potency and reduces the dose required. The newest of the PIs are lopinavir, atazanavir, and darunavir, which need only be taken once a day.

With this large selection of antiretrovirals available, it became possible to tailor treatment to specific clinical scenarios.

Enfuvirtide is a '**fusion inhibitor**', a twice-a-day injection that works by preventing HIV from entering cells.

Another group of new drugs is the **CCR5 inhibitors**, more suitable for those in the early stages of disease.

Integrase inhibitors such as raltegravir specifically target the virus itself and block HIV replication. They are well tolerated but are prone to resistance if not taken regularly. Elvitegravir, a once-daily option, will be available shortly.

What are the principles of treatment?

HIV increases at a rate of approximately 10^9 viral particles a day. This rapid turn-over leads to mutations in the virus, facilitating development of drug resistance.

The most important aspect of treatment is *adherence*. A low level of drugs in the blood can lead to resistance to the drugs and failure of that specific regime. Studies have shown that adherence needs to be better than 95%.

> Good adherence means that the person has to take the right dose at the right time more than 95% of the time

CD4 counts and viral loads are measured repeatedly during the first 6 months, aiming to reduce the viral load to less than 50 copies/ml.

Are there side effects with treatment?

Any new drug can cause side effects—you should seek medical opinion if this happens. The aim of HIV treatment is to give a good and long quality of life. If side effects don't settle down or are intolerable (or are serious), the drugs can be changed. We usually find a combination for each individual, that, after a few weeks, has no or minimal side effects.

What does resistance testing mean?

This looks at an individual's personal virus to see whether it is resistant to any drugs. 'Primary resistance' occurs when a person is infected with HIV *already* resistant to certain drugs. The person from whom the infection was acquired already had a resistant strain of HIV. This occurs in approximately 8% of transmissions.

Every new patient diagnosed with HIV has resistance testing done to guide the choice of drug to be used if or when they need treatment. The test is also important when treatment appears to be failing. It helps the next combination to be planned accurately.

Should I take part in a clinical trial?

Most large HIV centres have their own research unit employing doctors and research nurses. Because we now have drugs that provide effective treatment for HIV, potential new drugs are *not* compared with placebo but with the best treatment available. New drugs go through extensive trials before they are used in trials involving patients.

Trials these days not only look at new drugs but also answer important and topical questions such as:

- How beneficial is treatment in primary HIV infection?
- What are the long-term effects of HAART?
- Do the newer PIs need to be given with NRTIs or are they effective enough on their own?
- What is the rate of heart disease in HIV-positive patients and what effects do HIV drugs have on this?

Also under investigation are potential HIV vaccines. These are both preventative, to stop the virus being caught in the first place, and therapeutic, to slow down progression of the diseases in those already infected.

Why would anyone want to take part in studies such as these?

Without HIV-infected people taking part in research, the HIV field would not have progressed so quickly in such a short space of time. As well as benefits to all HIV people, those taking part will have access to newer drugs, extra investigations, and (mixed blessing?) see their doctor more frequently.

Any proposed trial has to gain local ethics board approval. Developing countries are no exception and drug companies have to adhere to strict guidelines which include, for example, an undertaking to provide their drugs for the study patients, lifelong, not just for the duration of the trial.

Resources

http://www.bashh.org/guidelines HIV testing, the window period, PEP, syphilis and HIV, reproductive health, and HIV.

http://www.tht.org.uk The Terence Higgins Trust advises all groups of infected people on all aspects of HIV/AIDS.

Index